BASIC HEALTH PUBLICATIONS USER'S GUIDE

TO

DETOXIFICATION

Discover How Vitamins, Herbs, and Other Nutrients Help You Survive in a Toxic World.

SHARI LIEBERMAN, PH.D.,
AND JAMES J. GORMLEY
JACK CHALLEM Series Editor

The information contained in this book is based upon the research and personal and professional experiences of the authors. It is not intended as a substitute for consulting with your physician or other healthcare provider. Any attempt to diagnose and treat an illness should be done under the direction of a healthcare professional.

The publisher does not advocate the use of any particular healthcare protocol but believes the information in this book should be available to the public. The publisher and authors are not responsible for any adverse effects or consequences resulting from the use of the suggestions, preparations, or procedures discussed in this book. Should the reader have any questions concerning the appropriateness of any procedures or preparations mentioned, the authors and the publisher strongly suggest consulting a professional healthcare advisor.

Series Editor: Jack Challem
Editors: Karen Anspach
Typesetter: Gary A. Rosenberg
Series Cover Designer: Mike Stromberg
Basic Health Publications User's Guides are published by Basic Health Publications, Inc.

ISBN: 978-1-59120-154-0 (Pbk.)
ISBN: 978-1-68162-679-6 (Hardback)

CONTENTS

Introduction, 1

1. Why We Need to Detoxify, 3

2. The Detox Diet, 18

3. Antioxidants and B Vitamins: First Line of Defense, 26

4. The Role of Phytochemicals in Detoxification, 36

5. Help from N-Acetylcysteine, Glutathione, and Alpha-Lipoic Acid, 41

6. Milk Thistle—The Master Detoxifier, 45

7. Other Herbal Detoxifiers, 51

8. Staying Toxin-Free with Green Drinks and Fiber, 60

9. Our Toxic Burden, 65

10. Daily Detoxification Program, 74

Appendices

A. Measuring Toxic Exposure, 79

B. Detox Diet Grocery List, 82

Selected References, 84

Other Books and Resources, 86

Index, 88

INTRODUCTION

If you've picked up this book, you already know that toxins and germs are prevalent in our environment—in the food we eat, in the air we breathe, and in the products we use. You also know that these harmful substances can interfere with good health and cause a host of illnesses. Although the need to detoxify our bodies is especially important in this chemical-laden, modern world of ours, the need to detoxify has always been with us. In fact, detoxification is highlighted in the oldest intact text still in existence, the Egyptian medical codex, known as Papyrus Ebers. Dating back to the sixteenth century B.C. (over 3,500 years ago), this text suggests that poisonous substances that contribute to disease are produced by undigested food in the intestines. Even then it was known that what goes into our digestive system and how our system deals with it greatly affects the state of our health.

In the West, however, it wasn't until the nineteenth century that detoxification was recognized as a necessary tool with which to combat illness. And it wasn't until the twentieth century that the importance of dietary fiber to our general state of health and to the health of our intestines was brought to light by scientists such as T. L. Cleave, Trowell, and Denis Burkitt.

These scientists familiarized us with the health-related dangers of highly refined, ultra-processed diets high in sugar and low in fiber. This information started the dietary-fiber craze. Everyone suddenly wanted a clean and healthy colon. Even *Saturday Night Live* got in on the act with their 1990s skit about a fictional high-fiber cereal Colon Blow!

While it's true that getting adequate dietary fiber on a daily basis is of utmost importance in any daily detoxification plan, it's only one of many steps you can take to detoxify your body. As you'll learn in this *User's Guide to Detoxification*, there are many things you can do to achieve a cleaner internal environment and, ultimately, a better state of health.

Chapter 1 begins with an explanation of how our environment and, consequently, our bodies have become overloaded with toxins. It goes on to explain what natural detoxification is and who can benefit from undergoing a detox program. Chapter 2 introduces you to a detox-friendly diet and gives you some suggestions for making changes in your eating habits.

Chapters 3 through 7 take you on a tour of antioxidants, B vitamins, beneficial plant compounds, specialized supplements, and certain herbs that can help you clear the toxins out of your body and promote health.

Chapter 8 discusses "super green" drinks and reminds you of the importance of fiber in a detoxification plan. Then, Chapter 9 alerts you to the toxic dangers lurking inside and outside your home and how you can reduce their impact on your health. Finally, Chapter 10 wraps everything together with a quick-and-easy detox lifestyle plan (no Colon Blow required—*promise!*). Appendix A provides resources for measuring your toxic burden, and Appendix B contains a handy detox-friendly grocery list. Be sure to check out the other resources listed at the end of the book.

CHAPTER 1

WHY WE NEED TO DETOXIFY

We live in a world heavily burdened by environmental toxins. Ever since the industrial boom of the mid-twentieth century, our planet has become home to dangerous levels of persistent organic pollutants (POPs). POPs are toxins made up of organic (carbon-based) chemicals and synthetic compounds. These pollutants are practically everywhere—in our soil, water, air, food, and even inside our bodies. We are even exposed to toxins through the seemingly harmless products we use every day, including such items as cosmetics, shampoos, hair products, and household cleaners. These toxins are collectively referred to as "xenobiotics" because they are foreign to the human body and have the potential to cause harm.

According to *Your Health & Your House* by Nina Anderson, more than 4 million new chemicals have been created since 1915. Clearly, our need to clear the toxins out of our bodies—that is, to undergo detoxification—is great, especially in this day and age.

Detoxification
The removal of harmful substances from the body.

How Do We Get Exposed to Toxins?

Our main exposure to POPs is from the food we eat. However, people who live and work near direct sources of these toxins (for example, industrial plants and modern-day farming operations) are prone to exposure through skin contact and inhalation.

The "Dirty Dozen"

Of the many hundreds of POPs in our environment, the twelve most dangerous (the "Dirty Dozen") have been targeted for global eradication by the United Nations Environment Programme (UNEP) Intergovernmental Negotiating Committee for a Treaty on Persistent Organic Pollutants. These are aldrin, chlordane, DDT, dieldrin, dioxin and furans, endrin, hexachlorobenzene (HCB), heptachlor, mirex, polychlorinated biphenyls (PCBs), and toxaphene.

Aldrin is a pesticide used to protect crops from soil insects and is widely banned. Chlordane is a chemical used to protect crops from termites and is also widely banned. DDT is a pesticide used on crops for insect control. It was used on troops during World War II to stop malaria, typhus, and other diseases. Although it is widely prohibited, it is still produced and used, especially to control malaria. Dieldrin is a pesticide used to control disease-carrying insects; its usage is restricted. Dioxin and furans are industrial byproducts that are partially controlled. Endrin is a pesticide used on field crops and to control rodents and is widely banned. Hexachlorobenzene (HCB) is an industrial byproduct released when plastics are manufactured. Its use as a pesticide is widely banned. Heptachlor is a widely banned pesticide that is used against soil insects and termites. Mirex is a widely prohibited chemical used as a pesticide against various ants, termites, wasps, and bugs, and also as a fire retardant in plastics, rubber, paint, paper, and electrical goods. Polychlorinated biphenyls (PCBs) are widely banned industrial chemicals used in heat exchange fluids, paint additives, carbonless copy paper, plastics, and various other industrial applications and released as byproducts. Toxaphene is a pesticide used on cotton, grains, fruits, nuts, and vegetables, and to control ticks and mites in livestock; it also is widely banned.

More on Dioxins, PCBs and DDT

Of the toxins discussed above, the most well known and infamous would probably be the dioxin and furans, PCBs, and DDT. Dioxins and furans are dangerous chemicals created when chlorine is produced. Burning and processing materials containing chlorine, bromine, and carbon also create dioxin. According to Greenpeace, "dioxin and furans serve no useful purpose because they are pollutants." They were "first discovered in the wastewater of pulp and paper mills in the 1980s and can be released through the air and as solid or liquid waste from pollution control equipment." A variety of industries and processes give rise to dioxins and furans, including producing, using, and disposing of PVC; chlorine bleaching processes such as those used by pulp and paper mills; burning medical or household waste in incinerators; and various metal-working processes such as secondary aluminum, steel, and magnesium smelters.

New dioxin sources are being investigated, as scientists believe there are still some unknown sources. The United Nations has compiled a list of potential sources. In Australia, a new dioxin source was identified when Southern Pacific Petroleum and Central Pacific Minerals (SPP/CPM) began developing the experimental Stuart Oil Shale Project near Gladstone, Queensland. Essentially, the creation and release of dioxin remains largely unregulated in the Australia-Pacific region. The chemical industry, meanwhile, continues to argue that dioxins occur naturally.

Bushfires and other types of fires (landfill fires, structural fires, household combustion fires, and even cigarette smoking and candles) do produce dioxin, but the high concentrations of dioxins and furans measured this century can't be explained away by natural sources.

Greenpeace points out that, like other persistent organic pollutants, "dioxin travels far and wide, resisting natural breakdown processes, and climbing the food chain until they reach people, where they bio-accumulate (build up) in fatty tissue." Dioxin is known to cause serious health problems, even in small doses. A piece of dioxin the size of a grain of rice equals the annual "acceptable" dose for a million people.

Polychlorinated biphenyls (PCBs) are a very toxic family of industrial chemical POPs. There are more than 200 possible PCBs, which are usually light or dark yellow and range in form from gases to oily liquids to waxy or hard solids. About 100 of the chemicals from the PCB "family" have been produced for sale, according to Greenpeace. They can be used as coolants, lubricants, plasticizers, hydraulic fluids, and dye carriers. PCB is also created "unintentionally," as an industrial byproduct with absolutely no value. They are generated and released by incinerators, chemical manufacturing, and magnesium metalworking smelters. Another big problem is that PCBs don't break down or dissolve over time, because they are "chemically stable." When PCBs escape into the environment, they attach themselves to tiny soil particles and travel through the groundwater table or above ground on wind and water currents. PCBs are hard to destroy. They resist fire and can only be burned at extremely high temperatures. PCBs release dangerous dioxin when they are burned, because they contain chlorine. Although Australia has proposed to remove and destroy all of their PCB stockpiles by the end of 2009, the PCB problem has not been adequately addressed globally.

Some insecticides have been banned due to their adverse effects on animals or humans. DDT is an example of a heavily used and misused pesticide. One of the better-known repurcussions of the use of DDT is the reduction of eggshell thickness of predatory birds. The shells sometimes become too thin to be viable, causing falloff in bird populations. This occurs due to the process of bioaccumulation with DDT and a number of related compounds, "wherein the chemical, due to its stability and fat solubility, accumulates to progressively higher concentrations in the body fat of animals farther up the food chain," according to the *Wikipedia*. The near-worldwide ban on DDT and related chemicals has allowed some of these birds—such as American bald eagle and the peregrine falcon—to recover in recent years. Nevertheless, the fact that DDT is now used in some parts of the world to stem the spread of malaria has given this old environmental nemesis new life.

Volatile Organic Compounds (VOCs)

Also of great concern to the U.S. Environmental Protection Agency (EPA) are volatile organic compounds (VOCs). VOCs are chemicals that release organic compounds during use and storage, some of which may have short- and long-term adverse health effects. Organic chemicals are widely used as ingredients in household products. Paints, varnishes, and wax all contain organic solvents, as do many cleaning, disinfecting, cosmetic, degreasing, and hobby products. Fuels are made up of organic chemicals. All of these products can release organic compounds while you are using them, and, to some degree, when they are stored. They are often a factor in sick-building syndrome (discussed on page 8).

EPA studies found levels of about a dozen common organic pollutants to be two to five times higher inside homes than outside, regardless of whether the homes were located in rural or highly industrial areas, and found the concentration of VOCs in indoor air to be five to ten times greater than in outdoor air. During the application of carpet glue and indoor pesticides, for example, indoor levels of VOCs may reach 1,000 times that of the outside air. The EPA is also taking sick-building syndrome seriously as an issue of inside pollution.

Sick-Building Syndrome

The term "sick-building syndrome" (SBS) is used to describe situations in which building occupants experience acute health effects that seem to be linked to time spent in a building, but no specific illness or cause can be identified. The complaints may be linked to a particular room or zone, or may be widespread throughout the building. In contrast, the term "building-related illness" (BRI) is used when symptoms of diagnosable illness are identified and can be attributed directly to airborne building contaminants.

A 1984 World Health Organization (WHO) committee report suggested that up to 30 percent of new and remodeled buildings worldwide may be the subject of excessive complaints related to indoor air quality (IAQ). Often this condition is temporary, but some buildings have long-term problems. Frequently, problems result when a building is operated or maintained in a manner that is inconsistent with its original design. Sometimes indoor air problems are a result of poor building design or occupant activities.

Causes of Sick-Building Syndrome

The following have been cited as causes of or contributing factors to sick-building syndrome:

- **Inadequate ventilation.** In the early and mid 1900s, building ventilation standards required fifteen cubic feet per minute (cfm) of outside air for each building occupant, primarily to dilute and remove body odors. As a result of the 1973 oil embargo, however, national energy conservation measures called for a reduction in the amount of outdoor air provided for ventilation to five cfm per occupant. In many cases, these reduced outdoor air ventilation rates were found to be inadequate to maintain the health and comfort of building occupants. Inadequate ventilation—which may also occur if heating, ventilating, and air conditioning (HVAC) systems do not effectively distribute air to people in a building—is believed to be an important factor in sick-building syndrome. In an effort to achieve acceptable IAQ while minimizing energy consumption, the American Society of Heating, Refrigerating and Air-Conditioning Engineers (ASHRAE) revised its ventilation standard to provide a minimum of fifteen cfm of outdoor air per person (twenty cfm per person in office spaces) in 1989. Up to sixty cfm per person may be required in some spaces (such as smoking lounges) depending on the activities that normally occur in that space.

- **Chemical contaminants from indoor sources.** Most indoor air pollution comes from sources inside the building. For example, adhesives, carpeting, upholstery, manufactured wood products, copy machines, pesticides, and cleaning agents may release VOCs, including formaldehyde. Environmental tobacco smoke contributes high levels of VOCs, other toxic compounds, and respirable particulate matter. Research shows that some VOCs can cause chronic and acute health effects at high concentrations, and some are known carcinogens. Low to moderate levels of multiple VOCs may also produce acute reactions. Combustion products such as carbon monoxide and nitrogen dioxide, as well as respirable particles, can come from unvented kerosene and gas space heaters, woodstoves, fireplaces, and gas stoves.

- **Chemical contaminants from outdoor sources.** The outdoor air that enters a building can also be a source of indoor air pollution. For example, pollutants from motor vehicle exhaust, plumbing vents, and building exhaust can get into a building through badly located air-intake vents, windows, and other openings. In addition, fumes can enter a building from a nearby garage.

- **Biological contaminants.** Bacteria, molds, pollen, and viruses are types of biological contaminants. These contaminants may breed in stagnant water that has built up in ducts, humidifiers, and drain pans, or where water has collected on ceiling tiles, carpeting, or insulation. Sometimes insects or bird droppings can be a source of biological contaminants. Physical symptoms related to biological contamination include cough, chest tightness, fever, chills, muscle aches, and allergic responses such as mucous membrane irritation and upper respiratory congestion. One indoor bacterium, *Legionella*, has caused both Legionnaires' disease and Pontiac fever.

These contributing factors may act in combination, and may supplement other complaints such as inadequate temperature, humidity, or lighting. Even after a building investigation, however, the specific causes of the complaints may remain unknown.

VOCs in the Outside Air

VOCs are also a serious outdoor air pollutant. They are often divided into separate catagories—methane (CH4) VOCs and non-methane (NMVOCs). Methane is an extremely damaging greenhouse gas, one that contributes to enhanced global warming. Decomposing garbage in landfills and solid waste disposal sites emit methane gas, as do many household products. Within the class of NMVOCs, benzene is a known carcinogen that may lead to leukemia through prolonged exposure. Another dangerous compound is 1,3-butadiene, often associated with industrial uses.

VOCs also react with nitrogen oxides in the air in the presence of sunlight to form ozone. Ozone is beneficial in the upper atmosphere because it protects humans and animals from exposure to dangerous solar radiation, but it poses a health threat in the lower atmosphere by causing respiratory problems.

The Air That We Breathe

"Sometimes all I need is the air that I breathe," sang The Hollies on the radio in 1974. But how *is* that air, after all? Most air pollution comes from one human activity: burning fossil fuels—natural gas, coal, and oil—to power industrial processes and motor vehicles. Some of the harmful chemical compounds this combustion puts into the atmosphere include carbon dioxide, carbon monoxide, nitrogen oxides, sulfur dioxide, and (micro) particulate matter (tiny solid particles, including lead from gasoline additives).

Between 1900 and 1970, motor vehicle use expanded exponentially. Emissions of nitrogen oxides, some of the most damaging pollutants in vehicle exhaust, increased 690 percent during this period as a direct result. When fuels are incompletely burned, VOCs also enter the air.

In fact, the EPA has declared that "tens of thousands of people die each year from breathing tiny particles in the environment." A report released by the non-profit Health Effects Institute in Cambridge, Massachusetts, agrees with the EPA assessment. This study was reviewed by *Science* magazine and shows that death rates in the ninety largest cities in the United States rose by 0.5 percent with only a minute increase—10 micrograms (mcg) per cubic meter—in the environmental concentration of particles less than ten micrometers in diameter.

Studies in several large cities predict that the combined long-term effect will be 60,000 deaths each year caused by particulate matter. This is a staggering loss of life that can be eliminated by stricter emissions standards.

Water, Water Everywhere

"Water, water, everywhere, [. . .] Nor any drop to drink," said the ancient mariner in Samuel Taylor Coleridge's classic poem, *The Rime of the Ancient Mariner.* Strangely enough, we are in the same situation today, and our problem isn't merely seawater, as was the mariner's.

Clinical ecologists claim that foods are the most obvious environmental carriers of "toxins," and say that "anyone drinking unfiltered tap water and eating a typical Western diet is likely to ingest 100 synthetic chemicals daily," according to the *Encyclopedia of Healing Therapies* (1997).

These chemicals include pesticides and herbicides sprayed on produce, drug residues in the meats we eat, preservatives in processed foods, air pollution, household cleansers, and dust.

Reducing Our Toxic Burden

The EPA and WHO have estimated that there are between 560,000 and 810,000 synthetic chemicals in use today, with 2,000 to 5,000 new chemicals added to the market—and our environment—each year. We're exposed to a great number of these chemicals daily—in the air, in our food, in our water, in household and industrial products, and so on.

How the body deals with toxins depends on a number of factors, including age, sex, genetic factors, the health of the immune system, nutritional status, the presence of other disease, the pattern of exposure (frequency and level), and lifestyle factors (diet and exercise).

The Body's Detox System— Removing the Poisons

Although our bodies did not evolve to deal with modern-day toxic chemicals, the same system the body uses to render "natural" toxins harmless (or less harmful) in preparation for elimination is also used to deal with many of today's "Frankenchemicals," too, with greater and lesser degrees of success.

The term "detoxification" is used fairly often, these days, when referring to cleansing our bodies from whatever poisons (including pharmaceutical drugs) that have accumulated due to drug regimens, our pollution-choked environment, and chemically laced foods. Very often, though, little attention is given to how the body gets rid of substances it finds harmful to the kidneys, liver, and overall health.

The lungs, skin, gastrointestinal tract, liver, and kidneys are the organs of detoxification, jettisoning foreign chemicals, drugs, byproducts of our own metabolism, and excess (or oxidized) hormones, vitamins, minerals, cholesterol, and fatty acids. Unfortunately, many chemicals, such as DDT, are "lipophilic"—fat-cell loving. This means that they have a tendency to wind up in our fatty tissue and in the fat that is part of our cell membranes. These accumulated toxins are very difficult for us to break down and eliminate.

The body's detoxification system is made up of two phases: phase I and phase II. These phases are two separate systems that the body uses to get rid of unwanted foreign toxins, called "xeno-biotics."

In phase I, the body changes nonelectrically charged (nonpolar), nonwater-soluble chemicals into relatively polar (electrically charged) chemicals that can then be excreted. Our bodies use certain enzymes to perform this process, which is a type of biotransformation. These enzymes make up two systems: the cytochrome P450 monooxygenase system (the primary system) and the mixed-function amine oxidase system (the secondary system). The most popular gathering place for cytochrome P450 is the liver, although the kidneys and lungs are also significant locations.

Enzymes—The Body's Detox Engines

In phase I detoxification, our bodies' ability to use its detox enzymes is dependent upon our levels of certain minerals. For example, the enzyme alcohol dehydrogenase, which converts harmful alcohols (such as ethanol) to more manageable compounds called "aldehydes," needs to have enough zinc to perform this process. In the next step, the enzyme aldehyde oxidase, which needs adequate iron and molybdenum, changes the aldehyde into an acid that can easily be excreted in our urine.

The following nutrients help the body's phase I detox efforts:

- beta-carotene
- choline
- copper
- fatty acids
- garlic (due to its sulfur compounds)
- iron
- lecithin
- manganese
- magnesium
- milk thistle
- molybdenum
- thiamine (B_1)
- vitamin C
- zinc

In phase II detoxification, chemical groups are tacked on to chemicals to make them water-soluble, so they can be eliminated through the kidneys. The following nutrients (some of which are already listed as nutrients for phase I) assist phase II detox:

- B-complex vitamins
- d-glucarate
- garlic
- germanium
- magnesium
- manganese
- molybdenum
- N-acetyl cysteine
- selenium
- taurine
- zinc

What Influences Detoxification?

Our ability to get rid of or disarm the poisons in our system, or detoxify xenobiotics, is influenced by several factors: genetics, age, sex, and lifestyle habits such as smoking. Other critical factors include the actual level of toxin/xenobiotic exposure and the presence of specific dietary compounds. While we may not be able to influence all of these factors, we can certainly influence enough of them to make a huge difference.

Nature vs. Anti-Nature

It should not be a surprise that our best route to defend ourselves within (or against) a "toxic," largely synthetic, chemical-drenched "anti-nature" world is through nature itself, including herbs and nutrients. Is this an indication of the "wisdom of nature" versus the "follies of industrial progress"? Perhaps, but it's nice to know that we have a powerful arsenal at our disposal.

We have control over lifestyle factors such as smoking or excessive alcohol consumption, for instance—both of which get in the way of detoxification.

While we can't live in a bubble or all move to the Himalayas to avoid xenobiotics, we can take steps to reduce our everyday exposure to toxins, which is sometimes referred to as our toxic burden or toxic load. For example, some big steps we can take include moving to a less-polluted city; installing a solar-powered, wind-powered, or geothermal unit; and purchasing a hybrid or hydrogen-powered vehicle (when or as available). Other smaller yet important steps we can take include using an air ionizer, eating more organic food, and using more (or only) natural household and cosmetic products.

We should also try to limit our use of drugs—including over-the-counter, prescription, and recreational drugs. Any little thing we can do to reduce our exposure to synthetic chemicals adds up.

Working *with* the Body

In addition to the steps mentioned above, there are specific dietary tools, components, and nutritional compounds that are crucial to detoxification. These include:

- A high-fiber "detox diet," rich in cruciferous vegetables (such as broccoli and cabbage) and beneficial compounds (such as flavonoids).

- An array of specialized supplements, such as N-acetylcysteine (NAC), glutathione sulf hydryl (GSH), and alpha-lipoic acid; and key herbal supplements, such as milk thistle and *Picrorhiza kurroa*.

We need a regular supply of many of these nutrients and compounds for our bodies' P450 detoxification system to do its job well. We have the greatest potential to experience harm when the chemicals or toxins we are exposed to overwhelm our P450 enzymes—probably because we don't have enough dietary components to support the system.

There is an association between sluggish or incomplete detoxification and cancer, chronic fatigue syndrome (CFS), fibromyalgia, multiple sclerosis, lupus, rheumatoid arthritis, Parkinson's disease, sick-building syndrome, allergies, asthma, sinusitis, and other diseases.

The Gastrointestinal Tract and Detoxification

In addition to the liver, the gastrointestinal (GI) tract is also extremely important in detoxification. The first contact the body makes with many toxins is through the gastrointestinal tract. Over the course of our lifetime, the gastrointestinal tract processes more than 100 tons of food. If we think about everything we eat, drink, and swallow, our GI tract—like the liver—has an enormous job to do.

Gastrointestinal (GI) Tract
Also referred to as the alimentary canal, the gut, or the digestive tract, this is the system of organs that takes in food, digests it to extract energy and nutrients, and expels remaining waste.

We know that fiber is crucial to keep things "moving" smoothly through the digestive system. We have to help our bodies to make sure that bowel movements occur daily, to minimize contact with toxins passing through the GI tract. The GI tract also has its very own complex detoxification enzymes and systems to handle the huge volume of biomaterial it has to process. The Detox Diet described in the following chapter is designed to help your body perform this very natural, but very vital, final process of digestion.

CHAPTER 2

THE DETOX DIET

The purpose of the Detox Diet is to clean and purge the body of toxins through the consumption of a wide array of naturally occurring plant compounds in food. These compounds are critical for optimal detoxification.

There are ways to enhance the Detox Diet as well as the body's built-in detoxification functions. Here are a few of them:

1. Drink plenty of fluids (this aids the function of the kidneys, bowels, and skin).

2. Allow controlled fever during nonthreatening sickness do its job, which is to put the immune system in hyperdrive to get rid of infection (bacteria or viruses). We should try to lower a fever only when it becomes too high or lasts too long.

3. Maintain a healthy circulatory and lymphatic system, partly with regular exercise.

4. Maintain good digestion.

Digestion

Digestion is the process by which food and drink are broken down into their smallest parts so their nutrients can be used to build and nourish cells and provide energy to the body. The physical process of digestion is as follows: After food is partially broken down in the mouth, it passes through the esophagus to the stomach, where digestive acids help the breakdown process continue. It then passes into the small intestine where further breakdown occurs and useful particles are absorbed into the bloodstream. The particles that remain then pass through the large intestine and are ultimately eliminated in the feces.

Digestion begins in the mouth, when we chew and swallow, and is completed in the small intestine; the biochemical and enzymatic processes involved in these stages differ somewhat for various kinds of food. Interestingly, bacteria, which naturally live in the gastrointestinal tract, carry out a good deal of the actual chemical work of digesting food for us.

The Cornerstones of Health

The digestion of food and the elimination of waste products form the cornerstones of health. If this dual system is not working properly, the body can be deprived of vital nutrients and become saturated with toxins.

As Ken Babal wrote in *Good Digestion* (2000), "To rephrase an old adage, we are not what we eat, but what we digest and absorb." Babal pointed out that the "flip side of nutrient availability/absorption is how well we get rid of the waste products."

We should recognize that "cleanse" and "nourish" are the numerator and denominator of the health equation. Both of these processes occur within the GI tract, which is where, wrote Babal, "our fueling station and waste-management system is."

Fiber's Role in Cleansing the Body

When many people think of classic nutritional detoxification methods, juicing and fasting usually spring to mind. It is true that juicing and judicious fasting have long been recognized as tools that help us achieve detoxification, but these approaches are difficult to follow for many people. Also, these detoxification pathways do not necessarily offer more benefit than actually eating fresh fruits and vegetables.

In addition, fiber is a critical dietary component if we are going to cleanse both the liver and the GI tract, and it would not be consumed if we were just juicing fruits and vegetables. Fiber allows us to eliminate toxins and other xenobiotics through the GI tract more rapidly by making bowel movements more regular. Toxins are excreted in your bowel movement, so getting them out of your body as soon as possible is important.

Another potential downside of the juicing approach is that when you juice and remove the fiber from your fruits and vegetables, you'll wind up consuming a much greater amount of sugar than if you ate the actual produce.

For example, apples have pectin, a great source of fiber. If you eat an apple, the pectin slows the absorption of the naturally occurring sugar in the fruit, so you don't get a great surge of blood sugar that could cause the crash-and-burn sugar "ride" many of us experience after eating cake, cookies, and other junk. Apple juice, unlike whole apples, does not contain any appreciable quantity of pectin, so when you drink apple juice you can get a sugar "rush" just like when you eat processed sugary foods. By eating the whole fruit and the whole vegetable, you get *all* the benefits of that particular food, minus the quick rise in blood sugar. Also, by consuming the whole fruit and vegetable, you'll feel more satisfied and not feel hungry. This is a perfect way to detoxify your body.

Getting Ready for Detoxification

It's best to prepare ahead of time before you start the one-week Detox Diet. That means cleaning the junk food out of your house (not that you don't have any willpower—right?). You will want to consider getting rid of cake, candy, cookies, processed foods, chips—anything you know isn't good for you. Take this time to go off all coffee and alcohol. Both of these substances interfere with detoxification, since they need to be detoxified themselves.

The One-Week Detox Diet Do's and Don'ts

- Eat only the cleansing foods listed in Appendix B. If you like, arrange these foods into three meals a day, plus snacks.

- Eat as many fruits, vegetables, and salads as you like.

- Do not add any fats to your foods: this includes oils, butter, and margarine. You may use a little extra virgin olive oil.

- Keep it simple. You may use spices and herbs. Small amounts of low-sodium soy sauce, salt, pepper, vinegar, and mustard are allowed, but avoid mayonnaise, bottled salad dressings, and ketchup, which has a lot of added sugar.

- Drink at least eight glasses or cups of herbal teas, distilled or filtered purified water, or mineral water every day. This will help you feel full and help flush away impurities.

- Avoid coffee, alcohol, soda, sugar, artificial sweeteners, and caffeine-containing beverages, since these can adversely impact detoxification. If you have been taking a multivitamin-mineral formula or other supplements, you may continue to do so, but do not suddenly start to take supplements during this detoxification diet.

- Get plenty of rest and sleep because it helps with the detoxification process. The naturally occurring plant compounds in the fruits and vegetables will help accelerate the cleansing process. For the first few days you may feel a little more tired than usual, but by the end of the week you should feel energized.

- Do not engage in strenuous physical activity, even if you are used to it. You can do yoga and gentle stretching, go for a swim, garden, or take walks instead.

- First thing every morning, drink the juice of a half a lemon in a cup of warm water. This old folk remedy helps your gallbladder work more efficiently.

- If you get hungry, feel free to eat more vegetables or drink more herbal tea or water.

The One-Week Detox Diet Grocery List

The Detox Diet works best if you are using raw fresh fruits and vegetables. (See the detox-diet grocery list in Appendix B). However, you can lightly steam vegetables such as broccoli, kale, spinach, beets, and others that you may prefer slightly cooked. Just make sure you are also eating salad each day to get some raw vegetables into your diet. You can use garlic, lemon, herbs, and spices as you like.

You can also drink "detox" teas that are available at your favorite health-food store. These teas often combine herbs such as dandelion, goldenseal, and burdock root, among others, to help assist in detoxification.

Or you can blend your own detox tea by using equal amounts of any of the following: burdock root, dandelion, fennel, or ginger. Feel free to use the age-old remedy for detoxification—dandelion tea.

Eat the Colors of the Rainbow!

The more variety you eat, the better the Detox Diet will work. When you eat green, red, orange, yellow—many different colors—you get the maximum benefits conferred by consuming a wide variety of plant compounds, vitamins, and minerals.

Go Organic

It's best to use organic produce since this is a detoxification program, and the pesticides and toxic metals found on regular produce are some of the very toxic compounds you want to rid from your body. In addition to pesticides, toxic metals such as lead, cadmium, mercury, and aluminum enter the soil and thus become part of our food as well. After some fruits and vegetables are harvested, nonorganic fruits are treated with additional chemicals to "fast-ripen" them. As mentioned earlier, we are even exposed to PCBs and other toxic substances in our water, thanks to run-off from pollution. Some harmful pesticides such as DDT have been banned for use in the United States, but other countries still use them— these are sometimes actually made by companies in the United States and then exported overseas—including Central and South America. We import much of our produce from these countries, especially in the winter, so we're still exposed to these chemicals!

That's why we strongly recommend that you buy produce that is organic whenever possible. When you buy something that has been "Certified Organic," it indicates that the food meets a federal government standard. That means it is grown without pesticides, herbicides, or chemical fertilizers. In addition, organic produce has much lower amounts of toxic metals.

There is also growing evidence that organic plant foods are more nutritious than conventionally grown food. A 1993 article in the *Journal of Applied Nutrition* sampled produce over a two-year period. The items studied—organic pears, apples, potatoes, and wheat—contained on average 90 percent more nutrients than conven-tionally grown versions of these same foods. Another study demonstrated that organic pro-duce contained *six times* the concentration of antioxidants compared to that of conventionally grown foods. That translates to 600 percent more antioxidants!

If your produce is not organic, you can still reduce the toxins that may enter your body. Wash and scrub fruits and vegetables thoroughly under running water, or use a natural product specifi-cally designed to clean off pesticide and fungi-cide residues. Peel off the outer skin because it contains most of the residue.

How Often to Detox

How often you should do the Detox Diet will depend on your particular needs. Some folks like to do the diet four times each year, with the change of seasons. Others prefer to do it once a month. In our opinion, we feel that four times each year is enough to reap significant benefits.

Keep the Benefits Long After the Diet Is Completed!

After completing the Detox Diet, try to make sure to continue to eat as much organic produce and other foods as possible, including meat and poultry. Stick to leaner sources of protein, such as chicken, turkey, fish, and seafood. The best fish to eat is *wild* Alaskan salmon. It has the lowest lev-els of mercury and other xenobiotics. Smaller fish, such as sardines and herring, are also lower in mercury. Fish is also a great source of omega-3 fatty acids that are also important for detoxifi-cation. High saturated-fat diets are detrimental to detoxification and should not be followed; these diets can also interfere with detoxification. Avoid fried foods and charbroiled meats since this is also another source of carcinogens. Purified fish oil supplements can also be used to get substantial levels of omega-3 fatty acids, without the concern about toxins. Flax meal (ground flax seeds) is an excellent vegetarian, omega-3-rich food, and also provides the added benefits of fiber.

CHAPTER 3

ANTIOXIDANTS AND B VITAMINS: FIRST LINE OF DEFENSE

Anti-what? *Antioxidants!* Sometimes terms are so commonly bandied about that we lose the meaning behind them. It's really worthwhile to stop and look back to the roots of this word—to what is important about antioxidants, and why it is important. Back to what it means to us as we try to make sense of nutrition and its effect on optimal health. Antioxidants are the knights in shining armor of our detoxification efforts. Not only do they neutralize toxins (such as free radicals) released during detoxification, they also continually support and strengthen our cell membranes, and even protect our genetic blueprints (or DNA) from being damaged by toxic bombardment.

So, let's take a step backward to see where the whole free-radical theory began.

Understanding Free Radicals

A critical step forward in antiaging research was first introduced by R. Gerschman in 1954, and expanded on by Denham Harman of the University of Nebraska College of Medicine. Their research revealed how free radicals produced by the body affect cellular health and energy processes.

Although a certain level of production of free radicals is necessary to provide the biochemical power needed to produce energy, maintain immunity, synthesize hormones, transmit nerve impulses, contract our muscles, and for other bodily functions, excessive free-radical activity brings rise to attacks on our cell membranes.

These attacks lead to the creation of metabolic waste products, such as lipofuscins. An excess of lipofuscins cause a darkening of the skin in certain areas, which are often called *age spots*. These indicate an excess of metabolic waste resulting from cellular destruction.

Lipofuscins also get in the way of our cells' ability to repair and reproduce themselves (replicate); DNA and RNA synthesis; and protein synthesis, which lowers our energy levels and keeps the body from building muscle mass. They also destroy cellular enzymes required for critical chemical processes.

Excessive, or uncontrolled, free-radical damage can be prevented by responsible supplementation with antioxidants. Simply put, antioxidants are substances that interrupt oxidation reactions, and, in most cases, prevent them from occurring. Making sure we have adequate antioxidant protection is our way to put the brakes on premature aging and prevent a host of degenerative diseases.

The Long-Term Effects of Oxidation and Free Radicals

Is oxidation a bad thing in itself? No. It's part of the cycle of all life, and it affects both organic cells and inorganic matter. "Almost everything is gradually oxidized by oxygen: fats turn rancid, rubber loses elasticity, paper turns brown, and even iron gradually rusts in the air," points out William A. Pryor, Ph.D., a prominent antioxidant researcher at Louisiana State University. "Thus it is not surprising that the cells of all plants and animals show a continuous level of oxidative damage." The problem occurs when the cells in our bodies are experiencing excessive oxidative damage over an extended period of time.

Facts About Free Radicals

Free radicals are atoms or molecules that are unstable because they are missing an electron. In other words, while an oxygen atom typically has a nucleus with paired electrons orbiting around it, free radicals have an unpaired electron.

According to James W. Anderson and Maury M. Breecher, in *Dr. Anderson's Antioxidant, Anti-aging Health Program*, "It is the nature of these renegade molecules to seek out and steal an electron from any cell membrane or structure it strikes; the result is a cascading chain reaction of free radicals causing damage throughout the cells of our bodies."

How do cell death and tissue damage occur? Almost all of the oxygen we breathe is used by small powerplants within our cells called "mitochondria," which convert fats, sugar, and oxygen into the energy we need to function and live.

In this energy-producing process, a small percentage of the leftover oxygen loses electrons, and free radicals are created. The actions of these free radicals cause gaps in our cellular membranes. Calcium penetrates our cells through these gaps, resulting in calcium overload. This can lead to cell death, which, in turn, weakens organs and tissues.

Each of the sixty-three trillion cells in our bodies contains twenty-three pairs of genetic (DNA) strands. The free-radical onslaught "causes a typical human cell to undergo thousands of changes, or mutations, daily," Anderson and Breecher add.

Although each mutation can turn cancerous, this occurs rather rarely because carcinogenic mutations must occur on both strands of DNA at or about the same time. Since both strands of DNA are under bombardment by free radicals, damage on one or the other strand is usually repaired before the cancer process can begin.

The Antioxidants

The major antioxidants include vitamin A, beta-carotene (and other carotenoids including lycopene), vitamin E, vitamin C, and selenium. They are present in a wide variety of fresh fruits, vegetables, seeds, nuts, and whole grains.

The Dual Roles of Antioxidants in Detoxification

Antioxidants are used in the process of detoxification and also protect our bodies during detoxification. When certain xenobiotics are detoxified, the intermediate compound formed may be even more toxic than the original. In addition, the free radicals formed during detoxification can damage our tissues. Antioxidants quench free radicals so that they can do us no harm. They also protect against damage to our DNA, which is implicated most devastatingly in the development of cancer, as mentioned previously.

While we want to consume foods rich in antioxidants, we may get additional protection by supplementing with antioxidant nutrients. The suggested amounts are expressed as you would find them on supplement labels: in international units (IU), milligrams (mg), and micrograms (mcg).

The antioxidants (shown in Table 3.1) can often be found in multinutrient formulas including multivitamins and antioxidants. They can also be found as individual nutrients.

It is important to make sure that the beta-carotene supplement you take is natural and has mixed carotenoids for maximum benefit. Dr. Kedar Prasad, one of the foremost experts in antioxidants and cancer, analyzed a random sample of synthetic beta-carotene supplements and found that they had virtually no beta-carotene activity! There also is evidence that synthetic beta-carotene may block the absorption of natural beta-carotene and other healthy carotenoids. Other carotenoids such as lycopene and lutein have specific health benefits and roles in detoxification.

The same holds true for vitamin E. Natural vitamin E exists in eight different forms or isomers, four tocopherols and four tocotrienols. Each form has its own biological activity, the measure of potency or functional use in the body. What we purchase should be natural (d-alpha-tocopherol) vitamin E with mixed tocopherols. Other tocopherols such as gamma-tocopherol have their own unique health benefits and roles in detoxification as well. Synthetic vitamin E (d,l-alpha-tocopherol) has only one-eighth the antioxidant activity of natural vitamin E, and it does not have any additional tocopherols. You may also find vitamin E supplements that provide other important plant compounds such as tocotrienols that are also involved in detoxification and found in the same food sources.

TABLE 3.1. RECOMMENDED LEVELS OF ANTIOXIDANT SUPPLEMENTATION	
Supplement	**Daily Dose**
Beta-carotene (natural with mixed carotenoids)	11–25,000 IU
Selenium	200–400 mcg
Vitamin A	5–10,000 IU
Vitamin C (preferably with bioflavonoids)	500–2,000 mg
Vitamin E (natural with mixed tocopherols)	400–800 IU

B-Complex Vitamins

The B-complex family of vitamins is necessary for overall health. Moreover, they are *coenzymes*—the key components of enzymes in the body. Without them, detoxification is impossible.

While these nutrients may not be as well known

as vitamins A or C, they are certainly making a name for themselves.

The B vitamins work together as a team, which is why it is generally recommended that we take a B-complex supplement, rather than individual B vitamins. The main B vitamins used by our detoxification mechanisms include riboflavin (B_2), niacin (B_3), pyridoxine (B_6), folic acid (B_9), and cyanocobalamin (B_{12}).

Now let's get to know the whole "B" family—the B-complex and other B-like vitamins—and why they need to be on your "A" list of "must-have" nutrients.

Vitamin B_1

Thiamine (more commonly referred to as vitamin B_1) was previously known as the antiberiberi factor. Thiamine is a must for metabolizing carbohydrates, fat, and protein, and, thus, boosting energy. It supports the nervous system, aerobic metabolism, and is important for emotional balance. A deficiency can bring on loss of appetite, depression, memory loss, and sluggish thinking.

Vitamin B_2

Riboflavin, also known as vitamin B_2, is a water-soluble vitamin that promotes normal growth, facilitates the breakdown of fat, and aids the synthesis of steroids, red blood cells, and glycogen. Natural sources of vitamin B_2 include almonds, yeast, cheese, eggs, chicken, beef, organ meats, and wheat germ. Riboflavin also supports the health of the eyes and skin. The book *The Natural Pharmacy* (Three Rivers Press, 1999) mentions that this vitamin is also helpful in boosting athletic performance, as well as preventing mouth ulcers, migraine headaches, and cataracts.

Vitamin B_3

Vitamin B_3 comes in two supplemental forms—

niacin (nicotinic acid) and niacinamide (nicotinamide). It improves blood circulation by dilating arteries, which is especially important in the extremities and brain. Natural sources of niacin include cheese, beans, milk, meat, poultry, fish, eggs, whole grains, and brewer's yeast. Clinically, niacin helps maintain normal function of the digestive system, helps reduce cholesterol levels, and helps eliminate dizziness and ringing in the ears.

Vitamin B_5

Pantothenic acid was discovered in 1933 by Dr. Roger J. Williams and was found to be a true vitamin shortly thereafter. Its name is derived from the Greek word *pantos* meaning "everywhere," which is appropriate for this widely distributed vitamin. Common sources of pantothenic acid are cheese, corn, eggs, liver, meats, peanuts, peas, soybeans, brewer's yeast, and wheat germ. Clinically, pantothenic acid is necessary for the synthesis of red blood cells, steroid metabolism, neuron activity, and stimulation of antibody production. In his book *The Vitamin Revolution*, Michael Janson, M.D., states that a deficiency of pantothenic acid can lead to depression, fatigue, and insomnia.

Vitamin B_6

Pyridoxine (vitamin B_6) was discovered in the 1930s after a series of nutritional investigations of rats fed vitamin-free diets. The original compound that was isolated is pyridoxine, thus named due to its structural similarity with pyridine. Common sources of pyridoxine include bananas, carrots, nuts, rice, fish, soybeans, and wheat germ. Clinically, pyridoxine helps normal function of the brain, promotes blood cell formation, maintains the chemical balance among body fluids, and assists in carbohydrate, protein, and fat metabolism. Vitamin B_6 controls the absorption, metabolism, and conversion of amino acids into neurotransmitters, antibodies, digestive enzymes, muscles, and tissues in the body. The liver requires a lot of this vitamin to function properly. Vitamin B_6 also helps the body use nutrients from fats and proteins, strengthens the adrenal gland, aids in the breakdown of glycogen, increases the function of the energy cycle, and works as a mild diuretic.

Vitamin B_9

Folic acid, or vitamin B_9, is a water-soluble B vitamin that takes its name from the Latin word for leaf, *folium*, because it was first isolated from spinach leaves. Folic acid is found in brewer's yeast, liver, fruits, leafy vegetables, oranges, rice, soybeans, and wheat. Clinically, folic acid promotes normal red blood cell formation, helps to maintain the central nervous system, and promotes normal growth and development. Deficiencies in folic acid cause conditions such as anemia, weakness, lack of energy, paleness, mental confusion, and headaches.

Vitamin B_{12}

Cyanocobalamin, or vitamin B_{12}, is considered the most potent vitamin and is one of the last true vitamins that have been classified. The vitamin was discovered through studies of pernicious anemia. This vitamin is not available from plant sources. Animal sources in-clude beef, liver, blue cheese, eggs, fish, milk, and milk products. Clinically, cyanocobalamin works to promote normal growth and development, helps with certain types of nerve dam- age, and treats pernicious anemia.

> **Pernicious Anemia**
> *A condition that begins with megaloblastic anemia and leads to an irreversible degeneration of the central nervous system.*

Other B-Vitamin-Like Substances

* **Inositol.** Inositol is a simple carbohydrate that

was originally thought to be a B vitamin. Inositol is metabolized in the body into phosphatidylinositol, which then acts as a second messenger system to stimulate the release of calcium. Major sources of inositol include beans, citrus fruit, nuts, rice, veal, pork, and wheat germ. Involved in immunity, liver function, and cell membrane health, this compound has been used to help lower cholesterol levels, improve injured skin, and protect the heart. Inositol has also been implicated in improving the transmission of neural signals in individuals afflicted with diabetic nerve damage and numbness.

- **Choline.** Choline was classified as an essential B vitamin for the first time in 1998. Among other things, it is important for liver function, heart health, achieving optimal physical performance, and memory.

- **Biotin.** It took nearly forty years of research after biotin's initial discovery for it to be fully recognized as a vitamin. Its roles, according to Burt Berkson, M.D., Ph.D., include breaking down fats and creating new ones, constructing proteins from amino acids, and helping to manufacture certain building blocks of genes.

One of the best ways to be sure you're getting enough B vitamins is to take a B-complex supplement. If individual B vitamins are needed over and above this, this supplement will help to keep the whole "B family" in balance for greater overall physical, emotional, and mental health.

B Vitamins—Mandatory for Detoxification

As we've noted, B vitamins are generally found in whole grains (such as wheat, rice, oats, and rye), green leafy vegetables, eggs, nuts, beans, meats, poultry, and fish. Most of the B vitamins are removed when grains are refined into white flour and white rice. Although many white flour products are considered "enriched" because a few nutrients were replaced, the fact of the matter is that the vast majority of nutrients, plant compounds, and fiber have been removed.

While B vitamins should be consumed through your normal diet, you can also take a supplement to be sure you receive higher levels. B-complex and multivitamin supplements often provide at least 25 mg of many B vitamins including thiamine (B_1), and some also include pantothenic acid, biotin, choline, inositol, and PABA (para-aminobenzoic acid). (Folic acid and vitamin B_{12} are offered in mcg rather than mg in all supplements.) A deficiency or insufficiency of vitamins B_2, B_3, B_6, B_{12}, or folic acid can adversely effect your detoxification efforts.

CHAPTER 4

THE ROLE OF PHYTOCHEMICALS IN DETOXIFICATION

People once believed that vitamins, minerals, and fiber were the only healthful things we could obtain from fruits and vegetables. Not so. A dizzying variety of natural plant compounds, called "phytochemicals," have been discovered, with more being discovered each year. At a press conference held at the American Institute for Cancer Research (AICR), researchers presented reports on how individual phytochemicals seem to protect against different types of cancer, a disease with which toxins are significantly associated.

Phytochemical

Also called a "phytonutrient." Any chemical derived from a plant source, usually with health-promoting properties.

Phytochemicals and Cancer Risk

Let's take a quick look at some of the researched phytochemicals and their cancer-protective properties. Indoles, for example, are found in cruciferous vegetables, such as broccoli, cauliflower, cabbage, Brussels sprouts, and mustard greens. It has been suggested that indoles may stimulate enzymes in women that modulate estrogen and detoxify toxins found in foods, protecting against breast cancer development.

Isoflavones are associated with tofu, soy milk, beans, peas, and peanuts. They have been shown to inhibit estrogen receptors and destroy cancer gene enzymes, thereby inhibiting cancer cell growth and division. In a study by Aedin Cassidy that appeared in *The American Journal of Clinical Nutrition*, six premenopausal women were given 60 grams per day of soy protein, containing 45 mg of isoflavones, for a one-month period. Alterations in menstruation (delay), suppression of mid-cycle peaks in luteinizing hormone and follicle-stimulating hormone, and other indicators produced results similar to that of tamoxifen, an antiestrogen used as a preventative for women at high risk of developing breast cancer. The authors of this study stated that "the results may explain the reason for the low incidence of breast cancer and its correlation with a high soy intake in Japanese and Chinese women."

However, some studies suggest that fermented soy products (such as tempeh) and other sources of phytoestrogens (such as flaxseed) may be better for women than unfermented soy products (such as soymilk).

Lignans found in flaxseed, walnuts, and fatty fish also appear to block hormones that cause cancer spread, such as estrogen and prostaglandins. Polyacetylene, known to be present in parsley, destroys benzopyrene, a potent cancer-causer. The herb, rosemary, is graced with quinones, which are nonenzymatic biological antioxidants said to block carcinogens and cocarcinogens. Sterols in cucumber skin lower cholesterol and triterpenoids in licorice slow down rapidly growing cells, such as cancer cells.

Polyphenols found in green tea and artichokes may also offer protection from cancer. Hasan Mukhtar, at Case Western Reserve University, looked at skin cancer and polyphenols isolated from green tea leaves. The data "suggest that green tea possesses significant chemopreventive effects against each stage of carcinogenesis" and may be useful against the inflammatory reactions associated with exposure to chemical tumor-promoters and solar radiation.

Clearly, vegetable and botanical phytochemicals appear to play a major role in decreasing the risk of cancer development at every stage—from cell penetration by cancer-causing agents to the abnormal cell production that is diagnosed as cancer, according to John Potter, Ph.D., M.D., program head of the Cancer Prevention Research Program at Seattle's Fred Hutchinson Cancer Research Center.

Plant Foods After the Detox Diet

Even after you're finished with the plant-based Detox Diet, you'll still want to eat a significant number of foods that help fuel your body's detoxification efforts on a daily basis. The more you incorporate these foods into your diet, the more optimally your body will be able to detoxify xenobiotics.

As mentioned earlier, there are many classes of detox-friendly compounds in plant foods. Let's take a closer look at some beneficial phytonutrients as well as the all-important plant nutrient, fiber.

Lignans help metabolize estrogen to its safest form. Lignans also prevent xenoestrogens from binding to estrogen receptor sites, which are implicated in cancer. They're found in beans, lentils, and flax.

Xenohormones
Pollutants such as pesticides, fungicides, and chemical fertilizers that originate outside the body and have hormone-like and estrogenlike actions within the body.

Indoles are crucial compounds that detoxify many environmental chemicals, including xenohormones found in pesticides and plastics. Indoles are found in cruciferous vegetables such as cabbage, broccoli, cauliflower, kale, and Brussels sprouts.

Ellagic acid detoxifies a wide variety of xenobiotics, particularly those implicated in cancer. It is found in fruits, nuts, vegetables, and green tea. Glucarate, which is found in fruits specifically, helps us detoxify carcinogens. Quercetin is the major flavonoid in our diet. *Flavonoids* are powerful plant compounds critical for detoxification of many xenobiotics. They are also powerful antioxidants: Flavonoids have greater antioxidant activity than vitamin C or E, and also are synergistic with these vitamins, becoming more effective in their presence. They also help convert estrogen to its safer form. Flavonoids are found in fresh fruits, vegetables, nuts, seeds, grains, legumes (including soy), extra virgin olive oil, green tea, and red wine.

Monoterpenes help to detoxify a vast array of xenobiotics. D-limonene, found in lemons, may well be the most studied monoterpene. Thiols, found in onions, garlic, and leeks, are plant compounds that detoxify a wide variety of xenobiotics, specifically mercury. Sulforaphanes are extremely important plant compounds in the battle against toxins. They are found in foods such as broccoli, mustard, and kale.

And, as you know, fiber is an important component of plant food that helps the body digest food better and more quickly. The term "fiber" refers to carbohydrates that cannot be digested. Fiber is present in all food plants, including fruits, vegetables, grains, and legumes. However, not all fiber is the same, and there are a number of ways to categorize it. One method is by the source or origin of the fiber; for example, fiber from grains is referred to as *cereal fiber.* Another way of categorizing fiber is by how easily it dissolves in water. Soluble fiber (from oatmeal, oat bran, nuts, and legumes) partially dissolves in water. Insoluble fiber (from whole grains and wheat bran) does not dissolve in water. Fiber can bind to some xenobiotics, thus shortening our exposure to xenobiotics passing through our GI tract.

Spice Up Your Detoxification

Many spices and herbs contain phytochemicals that are important for detoxification. In addition to garlic and onions, cilantro is an excellent herb that specifically detoxifies mercury as well as other xenobiotics. Curcumin, the active compound in turmeric, has anti-inflammatory and antioxidant effects, and a few studies have associated a lower incidence of colorectal cancer with high consumption of curcumin-rich foods.

A Serious Problem

Government surveys known as the NHANES (National Health and Nutrition Examination Surveys) have shown that on any given day an average American doesn't eat a *single* fruit or vegetable. Where on earth are they going to get any of these important plant compounds required by the body to detoxify xenobiotics? From soda? We don't think so. How about from a hamburger and fries? Hardly. So you can start to see the problem. We are exposed to more and more xenobiotics and are eating less and less of the foods necessary to detoxify these chemicals.

Toxin/xenobiotic overload is a real and serious worldwide problem. That's why it's imperative to take steps to minimize your exposure to toxins on a daily basis. Be sure to eat foods, herbs, and spices that help detoxify your body, and consider some specialized dietary supplements that can also be of tremendous benefit.

CHAPTER 5

HELP FROM N-ACETYLCYSTEINE, GLUTATHIONE, AND ALPHA-LIPOIC ACID

Unlike the antioxidants and B vitamins discussed in Chapter 4, this chapter discusses certain supplements we can make in our bodies when our diets provide optimal amounts of specific amino acids and other nutrients. N-acetylcysteine (NAC), glutathione (GSH), and alpha-lipoic acid (ALA) are powerful antioxidants that are also very important for detoxification. Whether or not you should supplement your diet with any or all of these nutrients will depend upon your level of toxicity. You may consider one or more of them if you have confirmed toxicity through a toxic metal analysis (see Appendix A), or if you have a condition or an environmental situation associated with toxicity as described in previous chapters.

N-Acetylcysteine (NAC)

NAC is the precursor to GSH. It has been in clinical use for more than thirty years. NAC enhances detoxification by the liver, and can prevent mutagenic and carcinogenic substances from becoming even more toxic during the process of detoxification. It is a powerful antioxidant that can also protect cells against damage caused by free radicals and oxidative stress. Data suggest that NAC may inhibit lung damage caused by secondhand smoke. Several experimental studies have shown that NAC is protective against many compounds that can cause severe and often fatal liver damage.

The most studied clinical application for NAC

is in acetaminophen (Tylenol) overdose. Liver damage usually develops within several hours of overdose due to metabolites that are very toxic and subsequently damage the liver. NAC is the antidote of choice and is used in clinical medicine to rescue people from overdose and prevent permanent liver damage. A recent study published in *The Archives of Internal Medicine* revealed that Tylenol, when used over a very long period of time, can significantly raise the risk of kidney impairment. Women who had taken between 1,500 and 9,000 tablets over their lifetimes raised their risk of kidney impairment by 64 percent. For those who took more than 9,000 tablets, the risk more than doubled.

NAC may also have a role in the prevention of cancer. Experimentally induced DNA damage by a wide variety of carcinogens can be completely blocked by NAC. It has also been shown to protect against mutation caused by various xenobiotics and to reduce the incidence of several experimentally induced cancers.

NAC is an excellent chelating agent for heavy metals such as mercury, arsenic, and cadmium, and should be considered with heavy metal toxicity. A large part of NAC's action is due to its ability to replenish GSH.

Glutathione (GSH)

GSH is actually a tripeptide made up of the amino acids gamma-glutamic acid, cysteine, and glycine. GSH is used to prevent oxidative stress in most cells and helps to trap free radicals that can damage DNA and RNA. There is a direct correlation with the speed of aging and the reduction of glutathione concentrations in intracellular fluids. As people grow older, glutathione levels drop, and the ability to detoxify free radicals decreases. NAC is the precursor to GSH and can generally replenish it when it is depleted by xenobiotic exposure. However, GSH also has its own unique properties under certain conditions. Supplementation with GSH should be considered along with NAC with more severe heavy metal toxicity and other known xenobiotic exposures. It also plays an important role similar to that of NAC in detoxification. It is the most important intracellular antioxidant, protecting against cellular damage from toxins.

Precursor
A substance from which another usually more active or mature substance is formed in biological processes, especially metabolism. For instance, beta-carotene is a precursor to vitamin A.

Alpha-Lipoic Acid (ALA)

ALA is also a very potent antioxidant, like NAC and GSH. Most famous because it is an antioxidant that is both fat- and water-soluble, alpha-lipoic acid is a vitamin-like nutrient that is able to inactivate free-radical toxins in our muscles, internal organs, fatty tissues, and brain. Besides being a superb antioxidant itself, ALA recycles worn-out vitamin C, vitamin E, and glutathione, and makes them useful again. Its ability to work in both fatty and watery environments enables it to protect all parts of a cell from free-radical damage.

ALA can also chelate cadmium and mercury and should be considered with more severe heavy metal and other xenobiotic toxicity. Chelation therapy is used as a treatment for acute mercury, arsenic, lead, plutonium, and other forms of heavy metal poisoning. Chelating agents were introduced into medicine as a result of the use of poison gas warfare in World War I. Chelating agents bind with metallic ions so that the offending ion is held by several chemical bonds, thus rendering it much less chemically reactive and allowing the ion to be excreted harmlessly.

When to Consider Supplementation

Not everyone needs additional NAC, GSH, or ALA. Need depends upon several factors, including:

If you have heavy metal toxicity. With more mild mercury toxicity, NAC and/or ALA would be sufficient. With more severe heavy metal toxicity, NAC, ALA, and GSH should be considered. Your healthcare practitioner can assist you by providing testing for heavy metals (see Appendix A).

If you have certain diseases. Neurological diseases such as Parkinson's and Alzheimer's disease, chronic fatigue syndrome, fibromyalgia, multiple chemical sensitivities, asthma, sinusitis, allergies, rhinitis, autoimmune diseases such as multiple sclerosis and lupus, sick-building syndrome, or cancer may be caused and/or exacerbated by xenobiotic exposure. However, if you are under the care of a physician for any medical condition, check with your physician before taking these supplements.

If you are heavily toxified. If you feel toxic or know that you have been overloaded with xenobiotics that may be causing symptoms, you may want to consider these nutrients at least in the short term, until symptoms such as allergies, asthma, rhinitis, or headaches start to subside. Low immune-system function may also be a consequence of xenobiotic overload. You may also consider taking these supplements for three months for a more thorough detoxification, or quarterly (four times each year) for one month.

TABLE 5.1. RECOMMENDED LEVELS OF SUPPLEMENTATION	
Supplement	**Daily Dose**
Alpha-lipoic acid	300–600 mg
Glutathione	250–500 mg
N-acetylcysteine	600–1,200 mg

CHAPTER 6

MILK THISTLE— THE MASTER DETOXIFIER

Milk thistle is "one of the most ancient known herbal medicines," Daniel B. Mowrey, Ph.D., wrote in his 1993 book, *Herbal Tonic Therapies.* In truth, milk thistle (*Silybum marianum*) has a long history of use for treating liver disease, dating all the way back to ancient Rome, when it was used by one of the most famous healers at that time, Pliny the Elder.

The milk thistle is an annual or biennial herb that flowers from June through September, according to *A Field Guide to Medicinal Plants: Eastern and Central North America* (1990) by Steven Foster and James A. Duke, Ph.D. Native to Europe, it now grows in Europe, Africa, Asia, parts of the United States (such as California), and in Mediterranean countries.

Although it grows throughout the United States and Europe, a great amount of research on milk thistle has been conducted in Germany. It is used extensively throughout Germany, Europe, and most of the world to treat liver toxicity and liver disease. Interestingly, it is also used in veterinary medicine to prevent and treat liver dysfunction in animals.

With the spines removed, the young leaves are sometimes eaten as a vegetable. Traditionally, Foster and Duke inform us, a tea is made from the whole plant, and is said to "improve appetite and allay indigestion."

The leaves of milk thistle have been described as "without downe, alltogether slippery, of a light greene and speckled with white and milkie spots and lines drawne divers wales," according to Geoffrey Grigson's *The Englishman's Flora* (1955).

Known Compounds of Milk Thistle

David Hoffmann's *The New Holistic Herbal* (1992) notes that milk thistle includes the following compounds: silybin, silydianin, silychristin, essential oil, and mucilage.

"At some point in time, milk thistle seed has been used in the treatment of gallstones; disorders of the liver, gallbaldder and spleen; as a cholagogue to promote the flow of bile [...] as a remedy for jaundice from any cause; for indigestion, dyspepsia, lack of appetite and/or digestive disorders; and to treat: peritonitis, coughs, bronchitis, uterine congestion and varicose veins," says Daniel Mowrey in *Herbal Tonic Therapies* (1998).

Milk Thistle and the Liver

As early as the twelfth century, the milk thistle plant was being used as a treatment for liver disease. In 1986, Varro Tyler, Ph.D., noted that silymarin was still being marketed successfully as a hepatoprotective drug to shield the liver from infections such as viral hepatitis. Very often used for the treatment of cirrhosis, hepatitis, liver poisoning, and chemical or substance abuse, Foster and Duke point out that "silymarin, a seed extract, dramatically improves liver regeneration" in disease and poisoning.

Milk Thistle's Antioxidant Properties

A large number of published reports "show that milk thistle seed extract protects the liver against the effects of toxins such as carbon tetrachloride, hexobarbital [...] thiocetamide and salts of rare earth metals," Mowrey states in *Herbal Tonic Therapies*.

Milk thistle can act as an antioxidant with

many times more antioxidant activity than vitamin E, suggests *AIBR Scientific Reviews.*

Compounds in the plant interfere with the formation of liver-damaging leukotrienes, while inhibiting prostaglandin synthesis during inflammatory reactions.

Laboratory experiments have demonstrated the protective effects of silymarin against both natural toxins, like those from carbon tetrachloride, a standard hepatotoxic chemical used in laboratory evaluation of liver drugs, and from the deadly amanita (death cap) mushroom.

An Amanita Mushroom Poisoning "Cure"?

According to a noncontrolled (for ethical reasons) clinical study by G. Vogel in 1981, forty-nine patients with death cap mushroom poisoning were under observation in Germany, Austria, Italy, Switzerland, and France. "Silybin was administered," Vogel wrote. "The results ranged from amazing to spectacular."

What Exactly Is Silymarin?

Silymarin is not a single compound. It is a mixture of naturally antioxidative chemicals, which used to be termed "flavonolignans," but are more often today called "flavonoids." According to Frank Murray in 1990, "meticulous research in Germany in the early 1970s isolated the active principles in milk thistle," as David Hoffman spelled out earlier.

Bioflavonoids act generally in the body to increase membrane strength and reduce membrane permeability. Silybin appears to act in this way

Bioflavonoid

Any one of a group of biologically active substances found in plants. Notable sources include red wine, green tea, onions, grapefruit seeds, apples, and other fruits and berries.

specifically on liver cells. The flow of chemicals across membranes is the major way in which the body's biochemistry works. Any substance that alters this flow can have profound effects.

Silymarin and Alcohol-Induced Damage

"Silymarin appears to be capable of lessening alcohol-induced liver damage when taken prior to alcohol consumption and is used clinically in the treatment of alcohol-induced liver damage," Rob McCaleb, president and founder of the Herb Research Foundation, explained in 1991.

In placebo-controlled experiments, silymarin has been shown useful in treating alcohol- and drug-induced liver disease. A study by H. Feher et al., in 1990, showed that six months of treatment significantly improved liver function in thirty-six patients with alcohol-induced liver disease.

Milk Thistle and Cell Membranes

Milk thistle appears to protect and heal the liver in several ways. Most important, perhaps, it acts directly by stabilizing and strengthening the cell membrane of the liver, and probably most other cells of the body. Supporting this concept is the finding that milk thistle extract and some toxins actively compete for the same cell-membrane receptor sites. That toxins are unable to affect cell membranes in the presence of milk thistle extract argues for the stabilizing action of these substances. The observable result is the regeneration of liver cells, indicating that milk thistle's compounds are excellent free-radical-scavenging antioxidants.

Milk Thistle—A Free-Radical Scavenger

"By combining our current understanding of the physiochemical properties of milk thistle, we can better understand why it can be a therapeutic substance in the treatment of liver disorders; milk thistle is a free-radical scavenger," Dr. Murray explained in *Better Nutrition* (1990).

"It interferes in the production of leukotrienes and stimulates protein synthesis," Murray added. It is suggested, in fact, that one of the ways in which milk thistle speeds up the regeneration of damaged liver tissue is by signalling for cellular protein synthesis.

Milk Thistle and Enterohepatic Circulation

Since toxins are continuously cycled "between the gastrointestinal tract and the liver," Mowrey goes on to say in *Herbal Tonic Therapies*, toxicity produced through what is called a "continuous enterohepatic circuit" usually takes quite a while to develop. When milk thistle compounds are administered, the enterohepatic circuit is interrupted. The primary absorption path of the toxins is now blocked, and their reabsorption is mostly prevented.

"Cells not yet poisoned are protected from damage from circulating toxins," wrote Mowrey. These damage-protected cells now "act as centers for the generation of new liver cells. With time, complete restoration of the liver is possible."

Silymarin is truly remarkable. It is safe and non-toxic, and has the ability to detoxify a wide range of xenobiotics. More important, it can actually regenerate damaged liver cells caused by xenobiotic exposure, as described above.

Milk Thistle Dosages

Look for standardized milk thistle extracts, usually in capsule form. Milk thistle should be standardized to contain 70 to 80 percent silymarin. The usual dose is 100–300 mg (70 to 80 percent silymarin) three times daily.

Milk thistle can be taken along with other supplements. Based on the available scientific evidence, milk thistle is just about the best insurance you can have to protect your liver as well as other cells and organs against toxic/xenobiotic exposure. Unlike vitamins and antioxidants that are required for detoxification, silymarin can enhance liver detoxification. In this extremely toxic world, we believe milk thistle is something you should consider taking on a daily basis.

CHAPTER 7

OTHER HERBAL DETOXIFIERS

Modern-day research has proven that there are other excellent toxin-defying, health-promoting botanicals in addition to marvelous milk thistle. These include garlic and a trio of Ayurvedic herbal preparations from India. Each offers special benefits that have drawn the attention of scientists and healers throughout the centuries. This chapter discusses the characteristics and effects of each of these plants, and whether they may be worthy additions to your detox program.

Garlic

In ancient Assyria, certain plant medicines were held in especially high regard. Not least among these exceptional plants was garlic (*Allium sativum*). Garlic, called *sumu* in Assyria, was thought of, says John Heinerman, Ph.D., in his now classic *The Healing Benefits of Garlic* (1994), as an "ideal treatment for getting rid of intestinal worms, encouraging proper kidney and bladder function, and alleviating diarrhea due to contaminated food or water."

Garlic was also used against poisoning from toxic mushrooms and plants, and as a liver-supporting detoxifier. In fact, over the last decade, some important studies (mostly using cell-culture and animal-models) have reinforced this premise.

In 1998, Drs. Zhao and Shichi, from Michigan's Wayne State University School of Medicine, set out to see what would happen when mice that received acetaminophen were either given garlic compounds diallyl disulfide (DADS), and/or N-acetyl L-cysteine (NAC), or no treatment. They concluded that treatment with both compounds "effectively protected the liver."

Another study carried out several years back by I. Sumioka and others, published in the *Japanese Journal of Pharmacology* looked at how extracts from aged garlic extract (AGE) protect the liver from acetaminophen. These researchers discovered that pretreating mice with S-allyl mercaptocysteine (SAMC), a specific compound unique to AGE, prevented liver damage in these animals.

A study (also in 1998) by F. Khanum and colleagues, in Mysore, India, looked at the effects of feeding fresh garlic or garlic oil to rats that had been given azomymethane (AOM), a cancer-causing chemical. The authors of the study wanted to see what would happen with the detox enzymes, in particular. The study concluded that long-term ingestion of garlic (twenty-three weeks in this case) reduced the toxic effects of chemicals, including cancer-causers like AOM.

Another study focusing on the effects of diallyl disulfide on different organs in the rat was performed by R. & C. M. Munday at New Zealand's Ruakura Agricultural Research Center in 1999 and reported in the journal *Nutrition and Cancer.*

The levels of two important detoxification enzymes, quinone reductase (QR) and GSH, were "significantly" increased in the test animals given the garlic compounds, leading the authors to conclude that garlic's activation of these enzymes may help with detoxification and possibly even shield humans from "cancer of the gastrointestinal tract."

Did the ancients know something about the detoxifying powers of garlic? It seems that they very likely did, and the body of modern scientific evidence is continuing to validate that knowledge.

Garlic and/or other detox herbs are helpful for the following conditions:

Amanita (death cap) mushroom poisoning
- *Picrorhiza kurroa*

Dysentery
- garlic
- slippery elm
- bayberry
- turmeric

Giardia infection
- garlic
- barberry
- bayberry
- echinacea
- turmeric

Worms
- garlic
- black walnut
- pumpkin seed
- pumpkin seed oil

For cases of food or chemical poisoning, overdose, and parasitic/bacterial infection, be sure to contact your physician and your local office of Poison Control.

Ayurvedic Herbs and "Untoxification"

In the Ayurvedic tradition of viewing the human being as a single unit, with body organs and other systems of equal value, the digestive tract and functions are seen as being of highest importance to health. The liver has a whole battery of functions, including the formation and excretion of bile, which is necessary for digestion; keeping certain nutrients and fuel, such as carbohydrates and lipids, ready for the body to use; manufacturing plasma proteins; activating specific vitamins; activating and deactivating body hormones; and detoxifying drug, chemical, and biological poisons, or toxins, that invade our bodies every day along with air, water, and food.

In 1997, coauthor James J. Gormley wrote, "An Ayurvedic physician would shy away from employing what we, in the West, would call 'detoxification.' This practitioner would liken detoxification to waiting until your car's oil is burning and running jet black, then doing an oil change and system flush. The Ayurvedic approach, on the other hand, is marked by what might be called 'untoxification,' a continual state and process of proper fueling, regular care, preventive maintenance, and tune ups, when necessary, so that detoxification is never needed."

Ayurveda, including the herbals of Ayurvedic medicine, recognizes that seasonal weather variations call for alterations of our daily routines, and that our bodies also undergo seasonal changes that require a modification of nutritional support to address them optimally.

When the winter chill arrives, the digestive and absorptive functions are well balanced and ready for the taxing seasonal demands of obtaining energy from the caloric value of food. Ideally speaking, in winter, the key is to eat a variety of foods, frequently and in small quantities, which will continuously support the digestive processes and the body's nutritional requirements. This is part of what might be called Ayurvedic untoxification.

The Catch? Reality

Ayurvedic medical texts, and formulary "recipes," revealed a realistic acknowledgment not only of nutrition's importance in maintaining health, but also of the likelihood that people, just like you and us, will fail to always maintain proper dietary regimens. The liver, the body's great detoxifier, will need a lot of extra help to deal with this simple reality. Single herbs and combination formulas need to be available to compensate for our nutritional falls-from-grace.

Enter three Ayurvedic herbs which are more

than up to the job: *Picrorhiza kurroa, Phyllanthus amarus,* and *Triphala.*

Picrorhiza kurroa

We might not have originally believed that a small, perennial herb, one which grows modestly in the Himalayas at an altitude of 3,000 to 5,000 meters, would be such a powerful player in the international medicinal botanical scene. But we would have been wrong if we hadn't realized it. In fact, extracts from *Picrorhiza kurroa* have been proven to be super-potent liver protectors and immune-modulators.

The bitter roots and rhizome of *Picrorhiza kurroa,* an important Ayurvedic herb, have been used traditionally for asthma, bronchitis, malaria, chronic dysentery, viral hepatitis, upset stomach, scorpion sting, as a bitter tonic to stimulate the appetite and improve digestion, and as a liver protectant (hepato-protectant).

Picrorhiza kurroa Components

Until R. P. Rastogi and colleagues published their powerful article on the chemistry of the roots and rhizome of *Picrorhiza kurroa* in 1949, the most up-to-date biochemical analysis of this plant was an 1890 treatise by Dymock, Warden, and Hooper!

Since 1949, Rastogi and others have isolated a number of compounds from the roots, including a glucoside (simple sugar plus alcohol), a bitter principle called "kutkin," a nonbitter compound called "kurrin," and other components, including vanillic acid, kutkiol, and kutki-sterol. It was later discovered that kutkin is a mixed crystal of two glucosides—glucoside-A and kutkoside.

Liver-Protectant Extraordinaire

In an animal-model study published in 1990, Floersheim and colleagues reported increased survival (protective effect) when doses of a commercial extract of *Picrorhiza kurroa* were administered before the deadly death cap mushroom was ingested. (The lethal effects of death cap mushroom poisoning are primarily due to massive injury to the liver.) Similar results were obtained by Y. Dwivedi and colleagues in 1992. When the extract was administered after ingestion, an "increased survival rate" was achieved.

Infection with Parasites

In a 1990 study, R. Chander and colleagues found *Picrorhiza kurroa* to have "significant protective and antioxidant effects in the liver" in experimental infection with *Plasmodium berghei*. In 1992, the same author reported liver- and brain-protective effects in a similar experimental model. Specifically, beneficial "changes in glutathione metabolism" were seen in the liver and brain, and reduced lipid peroxidation was also documented.

Chemical Poisoning

Extracts from *Picrorhiza kurroa* have been reported to protect the liver (and body) in cases of carbon tetrachloride poisoning as far back as 1969 (V. N. Pandey et al.) and as recently as 1993 (B. Saraswat et al.). This potent toxin is one of innumerable VOCs, that, as we've seen, are often added to commercial indoor pesticides (such as xylene and kerosene).

Paracetamol (Acetaminophen) Overdose

In a number of studies, including one done in 1991 by R. A. Ansari and colleagues and another in 1992 carried out by V. Singh and associates, significant liver protection was demonstrated when *Picrorhiza kurroa* extract was given before administration of the paracetamol (acetaminophen in the United States)—a common ingredient in many over-the-counter (OTC) analgesics, which can injure the liver if overdosed.

How Does Picrorhiza kurroa Work?

Frankly, nobody knows why *Picrorhiza kurroa* works as it does, although there are theories. R. Chander, one of the researchers cited above, suggests that the extract's primary components are excellent free-radical scavengers, and that this activity contributes to liver protection by reducing lipid peroxidation (a source of free radicals) and free-radical damage. Another possibility is the extract's ability to stimulate nucleic acid and protein production in the liver.

Phyllanthus amarus

Used in Ayurvedic medicine for over 2,000 years, *Phyllanthus amarus* is a small tropical shrub that grows widely in Central and Southern India. It is called *Bahupatra* in Sanskrit (and was once called *Phyllanthus niruri* in India). *Phyllanthus amarus* has big benefits for liver health and more.

This plant has been highly valued in a number of countries "for its curative properties; in India the plant is often used by traditional medical practitioners for a variety of ailments, including asthma, bronchial infection" and diseases of and injury to the liver, researchers L. Yeap Foo and Herbert Wong told us in their 1992 article in the journal *Phytochemistry*.

Phyllanthus amarus has been used for a wide array of indications, according to an interesting passage from Dr. K. M. Nadkarni's *Indian Materia Medica* (1954):

> The plant is considered [. . .] diuretic, astringent and cooling. A decoction of the plant is administered in jaundice [. . .] Whole plant is employed in some [. . .] genitourinary infections, [the] young tender shoots are [used in] chronic dysentery [and the] juice of the stem [is] mixed with oil in ophthalmia [eye treatments].

This liver-protectant/detoxifier is used in China, the Philippines, Cuba, Nigeria, Guam, East and West Africa, the Caribbean, and Latin America, and in recent years has been successfully used for such conditions as jaundice and hepatitis B.

Phyllanthus amarus Components

Studies have shown that *Phyllanthus amarus* contains alkaloids, lignans, flavonoids, fatty acids, and vitamin C, to name just a few of its components.

In a now-classic 1988 study conducted at Madras' Hospital for Children and the Government General Hospital (*The Lancet*, Oct. 1, 1988: 764–766), S. P. Thyagarajan and colleagues treated carriers of hepatitis B with an extract of *Phyllanthus amarus* for thirty days. Fifteen to twenty days following the end of supplementation, 59 percent of the hepatitis B carriers (twenty-two of thirty-seven) lost their carrier status, which essentially meant that they no longer carried the disease.

In 1990, Thyagarajan and Jayaram again joined forces in a study that examined patients with acute viral hepatitis B. Patients with acute viral hepatitis were given *Phyllanthus amarus* (250 mg, three times a day) for thirty days. The rate of "cure," or elimination of the virus, was 40 percent among those patients who received supplementation with this powerful botanical.

How Does Phyllanthus amarus Work?

As with *Picrorhiza kurroa*, no studies have clearly determined how *Phyllanthus amarus* works. One possibility is that *Phyllanthus amarus* may block the spread (proliferation) of the virus by directly blocking, or preventing, replication of the virus' genetic material.

Triphala

Triphala, which means three fruits, is a powdered

formulation from three different plants: *Terminalia chebula*, *Terminalia bellerica*, and *Emblica officinalis*. Traditional Ayurvedic practitioners refer to Triphala as a "good manager of the house," one which successfully attends to digestion, nutrient absorption, and body metabolism.

With a mild laxative effect that may be balanced by diet, this combination has been used for indigestion, constipation, and as an adjunct in ulcer healing, in addition to other uses.

TABLE 7.1. RECOMMENDED LEVELS OF SUPPLEMENTATION

Look for standardized extracts usually in capsule form.

Supplement	Usual Dose
Garlic	4 g of fresh garlic (one large clove) per day; follow manufacturers' instructions for powdered garlic and aged garlic extract (AGE) supplements
Picrorhiza kurroa	100 mg three times a day
89	
	200 mg three times a day
Triphala	250 mg two times a day

CHAPTER 8

STAYING TOXIN-FREE WITH GREEN DRINKS AND FIBER

If you are eating lots of fresh fruits and vegetables each day, then a "super green drink" is not necessary. But if you are often on the go, travel a great deal, or eat out often, green drinks maybe your best bet. Using this drink daily or even a few times each week will ensure that you get plenty of "green" such as seaweed, spirulina, kelp (ocean vegetables), cereal grasses like green barley and wheat grass, and even some green vegetables like broccoli and spinach. These drinks and supplements are easily found at your local health-food store and all have directions for use.

Ingredients in Green Drinks

Aside from the ingredients mentioned above, many of these super green drinks also contain milk thistle and many of the phytochemicals discussed earlier. They may also contain other antioxidant-rich fruit and vegetable extracts discussed in previous chapters. Seaweed is very useful for detoxification of heavy metals, in particular lead and cadmium. It also detoxifies a wide variety of environmental toxins, as does green barley. Some of these drinks even have acidophilus (the friendly flora) added to them to restore a healthy gastrointestinal (GI) tract. Some

Acidophilus
Short for Lactobacillus acidophilus; a beneficial health-enhancing strain of bacteria that have a symbiotic, or mutually beneficial, relationship with the human stomach.

of these drinks are made with mostly certified organic ingredients.

Some people prefer to use spirulina, green barley, or the same ingredients found in green drinks in tablets rather than mixing the powder with water or juice. These also work to detoxify a host of xenobiotics, and may be easier to use when traveling or may simply be more convenient.

A "shot" of fresh wheat grass juice is preferred by some for detoxification. Although this makes some wince, feel free to give it a try! There are many juice bars throughout the United States. that also have special preparations of green drinks for detoxification.

Fiber Rules

Remember in the earlier chapters we discussed that the bowel and GI tract processes tons of food, and it often the major site of toxic/xenobiotic exposure? This is why the one most important thing we can do on a daily basis is to eat a fiber-rich diet. Our government recommends at least 25 grams of fiber each day. This amount can be achieved solely through diet.

Foods rich in fiber include vegetables, fruits, nuts, legumes, and whole grains. The fiber content of breads and packaged foods are listed on the label, so this is easy to determine.

Fiber—A Good Carbohydrate

Fiber helps to regulate and promote healthier levels of blood sugar and cholesterol. It will also help with weight loss, because dietary fiber is not absorbed and fiber-rich foods make you feel full. High fiber intake has been shown to prevent certain cancers, heart disease, and diabetes, and is often therapeutic for these conditions as well.

Constipation

Constipation is often the result of a low-fiber

diet. Most Americans don't even come close to the 25 gram recommendation. If one is not having regular bowel movements on a daily basis, xenobiotics will stay in contact with the GI tract for a longer period of time, and thus have more potential to do harm. We want xenobiotics to move through our GI tract and be excreted on a daily basis. Certain types of fiber, like psyllium, flax, and oat, are water soluble and can trap xenobiotics in their gel matrix. This further prevents xenobiotics from causing injury to our GI tract.

If you are not getting enough fiber in your diet there are many fiber supplements to choose from, such as oat bran, ground flax seeds, wheat bran, rice bran, psyllium, pectin, and guar gum. Ground flax seeds (flax meal) taste great and can be added to food. Oat bran has a very mild flavor and can also be added to food.

There are many readily available fiber powders that can be mixed with water or juice. These can be found just about everywhere. There are also high-fiber crackers and chewable wafers that offer the same benefit.

There are some fiber powders that have additional ingredients for intestinal and bowel health, including acidophilus and L-glutamine. As mentioned, acidophilus is the "friendly flora" that keeps yeast and bacteria at bay in our intestines as well as in our urinary tract. L-glutamine is an amino acid that keeps the intestines healthy and both prevents and treats "leaky gut syndrome." Leaky gut syndrome occurs when the protective barrier between the intestines and the bloodstream is not able to do its job efficiently. When this happens, toxic byproducts of digestion as well as xenobiotics, bacteria, and viruses can more easily sneak into the bloodstream, when under optimal conditions they would be stopped. Leaky gut syndrome can increase xenobiotic exposure through the intestines. Certain medications and poor eating habits can also be contributors to this syndrome.

Other Constipation Relievers

If you are eating more fiber and still are constipated, drink more liquid. Water-soluble fiber in particular absorbs water and forms a gel increasing your liquid requirement. Approximately eight 8-ounce glasses of clean water (purified, distilled, mineral, bottled, etc.), herbal tea, or juice diluted with water or mineral water can help you achieve this amount of fluid intake.

There are natural products on the market for constipation, including senna and *Cascara sagrada*, but they can cause cramping and diarrhea in some people because they work by irritating the GI tract so more water flows into it, causing a bowel movement. The most gentle product we have found so far is the Ayurvedic herbal combination discussed earlier called "Triphala." It promotes normal bowel movements by gently stimulating peristalsis (the movement of food through your GI tract) and bile flow. It does not cause cramping or diarrhea.

Triphala is nonirritating and can be used whenever it is needed. It appears to also be nonaddicting. When used as a remedy for constipation, the general recommended dose of Triphala is to take one to four 120-mg capsules with warm water at bedtime. You will want to use the lowest dose needed, so it's best to start with one capsule and add another one every few days if necessary.

You may also want to consider an additional acidophilus supplement. Culturelle and Florastor are well-researched supplements, with more than thirty years of clinical data. Culturelle contains lactobacillus GG, which can help reduce yeast and control overgrowth of bacteria. Florastor's generic name is *Saccharomyces boulardii*. This reestablishes the friendly flora in the GI tract to inhibit the proliferation of *Candida albicans* and harmful bacteria. It is particularly effective against resistant bacteria caused by overuse of antibiotics.

CHAPTER 9

OUR TOXIC BURDEN

What we are exposed to on a daily basis is nothing short of mind-boggling. Use the information in this chapter to reduce your daily exposure to xenobiotics as much as possible. This is not a full inventory of everything you can be exposed to—that would be impossible to list!

A Sampling of What's in Our Water

We discussed water earlier, but we didn't specifically get into why drinking tap water can be hazardous to your health. Sewerage water is often recycled with a ton of chemicals to turn it into acceptable drinking water. The question is—acceptable for whom?

Here are a few examples of what you can ingest with your water: lead, mercury, cadmium, arsenic, pesticides (too numerous to list), DDT, chloroform, vinyl chloride, gasoline, xylene, toluene, benzene, herbicides, polynuclear aromatic hydrocarbons (PAH), nitrates, nitrosamines, asbestos, ethylene dibromide, and polychlorinated bipheyls (PCBs).

In addition to the xenobiotics listed above, here are some you probably never even thought of: residue from drugs like statins and other medications, and parasites such as *Cryptosporidia* and *Giardia*.

There have been numerous reports about the increase in drug residues found in drinking water. Incidents will continue to rise as America continues to use more and more prescription and over-the-counter drugs. While parasites exist in our water system, sometimes the load becomes high enough that there are outbreaks reported to health officials. According to *Consumer Reports,* cryptosporidium, a parasite from animal waste, entered Milwaukee's water supply in 1993. It killed more than 50 people, sent 4,400 to hospitals, and sickened hundreds of thousands.

Those are real, tangible reasons *not* to drink tap water. You simply don't know what you are drinking. There are many water purifiers on the market that take the vast majority of xenobiotics out of the water to make it safe to drink. They will list how much heavy metal, PCBs, and other chemicals and parasites are removed. Many of these use a carbon filter and/or reverse osmosis, while others can distill water and remove virtually everything except the water. It's really your choice, so it's best to compare pricing, the degree of purification, ease of use, and most important—taste of the water produced.

PCBs
Polychlorinated biphenyls; a class of organic compounds that enter the environment through use and disposal. Long-term effects remain uncertain, but many health conditions are associated with short-term exposure.

Consumer Reports Rating of Bottled Water

Consumer Reports published an article reviewing drinking water in August 2000. This report was an eye-opener for many bottled-water drinkers.

The best rated bottled waters were (in descending order): Volvic Natural Spring Water, Dannon Natural Spring Water (when bottled in PET but not in HDPE), Arrowhead Mountain Spring Water, American Fare Natural Spring Water (Kmart), and Albertson's A+ Natural Spring Water. Aquafina (Pepsi) and Dasani (Coca Cola) are purified water from municipal water systems.

The best carbonated water was Vintage Old Original Seltzer Water.

Mineral waters can have very individual tastes caused by the rocks the waters flow over in their natural environment. Vittel and Calistoga mineral water were less expensive than the others and were rated very good. The more expensive mineral waters, and the taste to expect, were rated as follows: Apollinaris Naturally Sparkling Mineral Water (moderate fizz, slight mineral and baking-soda flavors), Calistoga Sparkling Mineral Water (little fizz, slight earthy, mineral, and baking-soda flavors), Perrier Sparkling Mineral Water (moderate fizz, slight baking-soda flavor, trace of mineral flavor), San Pellegrino Natural Sparkling Mineral Water (a personal favorite—very little fizz, slight mineral and baking-soda flavors), and Vittel Mineral Water (no fizz, slight mineral flavor).

According to the report, water in PET plastic bottles generally tasted better than water in HDPE plastic, though water in HDPE is usually cheaper. The higher the rating of the plastic container on the side of the container, the less leaching of plastic will occur in your water. Our collective opinion is that since plastic is a toxic xenobiotic, your best bet is to drink out of glass.

Polyethylene Bottles

Polyethylene (PE) has two forms used in water bottles: HDPE (high density polyethylene), used for containers, plumbing, and automotive fittings, and PET or PETE (polyethylene terephthalate), used for making carbonated-beverage bottles.

Types of Drinking Water

The following are classifications of drinking water to help in your selection decision:

- **Mineral water.** contains at least 250 parts per million of dissolved solids—usually calcium, magnesium, sodium, potassium, silica, and bicarbonates. Minerals must occur naturally. Mineral water is typically spring water and can be sparkling or still.

- **Purified drinking water.** processed by reverse osmosis, distillation, or similar procedures that remove minerals and contaminants. The source of the water does not need be named and is often tap water or municipal water.

- **Naturally sparkling water.** naturally carbonated and often comes from a spring. Bubbles lost during treatment or collection may be replaced with the same amount of carbon dioxide the water held originally.

- **Soda water and seltzer.** not considered bottled water. The FDA regulates them as soft drinks, under rules less strict than those for bottled water, and some products may have added sugar, flavors, or salts. They're often carbonated municipal water, sometimes with extra filtration.

There have been additional brands of bottled waters brought into the marketplace since this report. Read labels carefully. Sometimes the name of the water sounds like an exotic place but what you are actually getting is purified tap water. Contact companies and ask for toxicology and contaminant reports. They should have these readily available.

Consumer Reports Rating of Water-Purification Systems

In January 2003, *Consumer Reports* rated home water-purification systems. For all filtering, water passes through a removable cartridge filled with a filtering medium, such as charcoal, that needs to be replaced periodically. There's a screw-on filter for just about every kind of tap in your home including the sink, showerhead, refrigerator water dispenser, under your sink, or in a basement.

Consumer Reports tested nineteen models ranging from $18 to $240. They purposely spiked the water with chloroform, a trihalomethane (THM), and lead, both widespread contaminants and health hazards at high concentrations. They then processed up to 240 gallons of water through each filter (less for carafes, or if a filter became clogged). The researchers also cooked up batches of cabbage-flavored water, ran it through each filter, and tasted the results to see how well the filters removed off-tastes.

All of the tested filters made removal claims certified by National Sanitation Foundation International (NSF). When any system claims removal of a contaminant, its label must be NSF-certified for that substance for you to know for sure.

The filter used by a particular system may be certified by another testing agency, or it may not have any independent third-party certification of performance. Independent testing and certification of performance further supports the validity of any performance claim.

The top-rated undersink model in the test was the Sears Kenmore 38460 ($80), which is certified to remove sediment, small particulates that cloud water, and cysts (formed by parasites). Two other undersink models, the Omni CBF-20 ($170) and Culligan SY-2500 ($180), claim to remove more: the pesticides lindane and atrazine, mercury, and asbestos. The Omni was ranked higher than the Culligan because it didn't clog as much.

Some manufacturers offer a variety of replacement cartridges, each designed to remove different contaminants. You can use those filters interchangeably if they're the same size and brand as the cartridge included with the filtering system.

Nearly all the carafes that sit in the fridge or

on a counter were rated very good or excellent at removing lead and chloroform, which is sufficient for most people's needs. You simply pour water into the top of the carafe and it's filtered as it trickles into the bottom reservoir. The sensory panelists found the Pur Advantage CR-1500R ($18) good and the Brita Classic OB01 ($20) very good at removing off-tastes.

Faucet-mounted systems screw directly onto a sink faucet. A valve lets you bypass the filter when you don't need to filter, such as when you are rinsing dishes. The cartridges in these systems last longer than those in the carafes, but still must be replaced four times per year. The rate at which they deliver water can slow with use. The only drawback is that the Pur Ultimate Horizontal FM-4700L ($43) clogged well before its cartridge's 100-gallon lifetime; it slowed to ten minutes per gallon by the time it had filtered 60 gallons in these tough tests.

There are other types of systems, such as under-sink and reverse-osmosis systems, that require professional installation. For any type of system that you choose, there are several certification and testing organization that can confirm the performance of the unit, including the following: www.nsf.org (National Sanitation Foundation), www.ul.com (Underwriters Laboratories), and www.wqa.org (Water Quality Association). These organizations can also assist you in getting your tap water tested.

There are also many water-purification systems on the market that were not tested by *Consumer Reports* that are offered through distributors. They may perform as well as or better than the ones that were tested. All units should have certification by one or more of the agencies listed, and all of the manufacturers should be able to provide specifics about the toxins and xenobiotics removed by their system.

Dangerous Products in Your Home

Unfortunately, the vast majority of commercial cleaning supplies are quite toxic. Your best bet is to substitute safer versions. These are available at the health store, but are becoming increasingly available at supermarkets as well. One chemical sometimes found in cleaning products, formaldehyde, should be avoided at all costs—it is a very toxic and carcinogenic compound. Here is just a sampling of some of the xenobiotics you can be exposed to that can be extremely toxic and irritating:

- **Mothballs.** paradichlorobenzene, toxic to the liver and kidney and irritating to the mucous membranes.

- **Dry cleaning spot removers.** perchloroethylene, when inhaled can be toxic to the liver and nervous system.

- **Chlorine bleach.** never mix bleach with ammonia or vinegar, since the resulting fumes can be highly toxic.

- **Drain cleaners.** lye and sodium hydroxide are very toxic to the skin and when they are accidentally ingested.

- **Oven cleaners.** lye aerosols are the most dangerous.

- **Glass cleaners.** ammonia and blue dye are very irritating. Aerosols are the worst.

- **Air fresheners.** phenol, cresol, ethanol, and xylene are toxic. Look for ones that state they are safe.

- **Germ-killing disinfectants.** cresol, phenol, and ethanol can all be irritating and potentially toxic. Formaldehyde is a potent carcinogen.

- **Mold cleaners.** phenol, kerosene, and formaldehyde are all irritating and potentially toxic.

Personal-Care Products

Among the most toxic ingredients in personal-care products is, again, formaldehyde. It can be present in mouthwash, cosmetics, perfume, after-shave, antiperspirants, dandruff shampoo, and spermicides. There are artificial colors in mouthwash, toothpaste, perfume, body lotion, shampoo, and other bath and body products.

Antiperspirants are among the worst offenders because they contain aluminum and are a major source of toxic metal exposure. Hair dyes can contain coal tar, which is toxic. Talcum powder may contain asbestos. There are safer versions of just about all these products that are becoming more readily available.

Other Toxin Sources in Your Home

- **Clothes.** Believe it or not, your clothing and the fluids used to clean them can be a source of xenobiotic exposure. Permanent-press clothing and fabric dyes contain formaldehyde, and synthetic fibers such as nylon, polyester, and acrylic are all plastics.

- **Plastics.** Plastics are a major source of xenobiotic exposure because they are everywhere. Here are some of the most toxic plastics, some of which are also carcinogenic:

  - Polyethylene: containers, wrappers, kitchenware, plastic bags, and squeeze bottles. Polythylene is toxic and possibly carcinogenic.

  - Vinyl chloride: the worst and most carcinogenic plastic.

  - Polyvinyl chloride: adhesives, containers, tapes, toys, beach balls, pacifiers, raincoats, boots—all release vinyl chloride, which can cause cancer, liver disease, birth defects, and have other serious consequences.

- Urea-formaldehyde plastic resins: particle-board, plywood, insulation, tissues, and towels all outgas formaldehyde.

- Flourocarbon plastic: tetrafluoroethylene is found in Teflon, nonstick coating, and ironing-board covers, and is very toxic and irritating.

- **Home pesticides.** Insecticides used in the house and the garden are generally very toxic. Many of them are potent carcinogens. Pyrethrum and other natural products are excellent alternatives.

It is in your best interest for your health and the health of the planet to replace anything you can with a safer, gentler more environmentally conscious product or alternative. It is virtually impossible to avoid all of these products. That's why we do want to consider supporting daily detoxification through supplements in addition to the Detox Diet.

CHAPTER 10

DAILY DETOXIFICATION PROGRAM

As discussed throughout this guide, there are some supplements that everyone should consider, and others that may be worth considering depending upon your individual exposures or conditions. The following information will enable you to put a daily detoxification program together to suit your specific needs after you have completed the Detox Diet.

Normal Daily Detoxification

For everyday detoxification, consider a multivitamin that provides antioxidants and B-complex vitamins at the doses recommended earlier. You can also match these doses with a high-potency antioxidant plus a separate B complex. Continue to eat fresh salad, vegetables, and fruits—preferably organic if possible. You may also consider the following:

- **A super green drink.** You can drink this daily or a few times per week to ensure your intake of a wide variety of detoxifying phytonutrients. This is especially good to use if you are not consuming enough fruits and vegetables on a daily basis to accomplish detoxification. These drinks are excellent to use for overall daily detoxification. Some of these drinks also have some fiber.

- **Milk Thistle, garlic, *Picrorhiza kurroa*, *Phythallus amarus*, and triphala.** Silymarin in milk thistle enhances detoxification of many xenobiotics and is one of the most liver-protective plant compounds. We would recommend these botanicals for just about everyone, as they all have excellent benefits.

- **Fiber.** If you're eating lots of fiber in your diet, then a fiber supplement is probably not necessary. If you are not, you should consider taking a fiber supplement daily or even a few times each week.

- **Phytochemicals.** You can get many phytochemicals in your diet—just by eating them. Chapter 4 deals specifically with which foods provide specific phytochemicals that detoxify xenobiotics. You should try to eat as many of these as you can on a daily basis, or at least a few times each week. Many of these phytochemicals are often found in the super green drinks. And there are "detox" supplements and teas that provide many of these phytochemicals as well.

Heavier-Duty Detoxification

If you know you are exposed to many xenobiotics, you may want to consider a more intense daily detoxification program. This would include the recommendations for the normal daily detoxification *plus:*

- **N-acteylcysteine.** NAC enhances liver detoxification and is very protective against carcinogens and heavy metals. It can prevent and reduce liver injury from medications. There is also evidence that it may also protect the kidneys and lung from xenobiotic toxicity as well.

- **Alpha-lipoic acid.** This is a very powerful antioxidant. The only issue is that it is expensive. Like NAC and milk thistle, it can increase levels of glutathione. It should definitely be considered in cases of heavy metal toxicity, especially mercury.

- **Glutathione.** Since NAC, milk thistle, and ALA can enhance GSH levels, taking GSH supplements may not be necessary for most people. You may want to consider taking an additional GSH supplement if tests reveal a rather high xenobiotic load (see Appendix A). You may also want to consider all three of these detoxifiers if you suffer from illness such as chronic fatigue syndrome, fibromyalgia, multiple chemical sensitivities, asthma, sinusitis, allergies, rhinitis, autoimmune diseases such as multiple sclerosis and lupus, sick-building syndrome, headaches, or arthritis.

If your pocketbook permits, it is perfectly fine to take both NAC and ALA on a daily basis. Many practitioners will recommend these supplements preventively to enhance detoxification.

The Mighty Sauna

The sauna or Finnish bath has a very long history of use, and its value is corroborated by scientific studies. It is used throughout Europe and is becoming more common in the United States since it has been shown to detoxify many xenobiotics such as PCBs, heavy metals, and industrial chemicals. The high sauna temperature stimulates lipolysis and enhances the excretion of xenobiotics that are stored in this tissue. Xenobiotics are excreted via sweat. It is also a good idea to use a loofa after a sauna and to make sure that you rinse and wash your skin thoroughly.

Lipolysis *The breakdown of stored body fat.*

The Detoxification Experience

After detoxification, especially after the Detox Diet, you may experience increased energy, mental clarity, better sleep, and an alleviation of various symptoms.

Remember that anything you can do to reduce your overall exposure is important. We cannot live in a bubble, nor would we want to, but we should become more politically proactive in cleaning up our environment. It is not only affecting our health, but wildlife is being seriously affected as well. The good news is that we do have the ability to protect ourselves by making sure that we are detoxifying toxins and xenobiotics 24/7.

MEASURING TOXIC EXPOSURE

While we can't test for all xenobiotic exposure, there are testing laboratories that can give us some important information. Please be advised that all of these laboratories require tests be ordered by a licensed, healthcare provider. The laboratories will be able to provide you with professionals in your area who can provide this testing.

Laboratories Providing Serum Tests for Pesticides and Solvents

These laboratories require blood samples in order to perform their tests. They are listed in alphabetical order.

Accu-Chem Laboratories
990 N Bowser Road, Suite 800
Richardson, TX 75081
Tel: 800-451-0116

National Medical Services
3701 Welsh Road
Willow Grove, PA 19090
Tel: 800-522-6671

Pacific Toxicology Laboratories
6160 Variel Avenue
Woodland Hills, CA 91367
Tel: 800-328-6942

Laboratories Providing Tests for Heavy Metals

These laboratories offer several ways to assess heavy metal exposure. Hair analysis is the least invasive and expensive, but it is the least accurate compared to other methods. It is not recommended if you use hair color, perms, or relaxers, or dandruff shampoos since all these can directly influence the content of the hair. Hair analysis can still be useful to determine overall toxic metal exposure. However, it is not permitted in New York.

These laboratories can also assess heavy metal exposure through both six-hour and twenty-four-hour provocative urine tests. You are given a chelating agent that pulls heavy metals (and also essential minerals) out of your tissues so they are excreted in your urine. Your kidney function must be evaluated before you can take this test. Another test is a stool test that can also assess heavy metal exposure. The laboratories are listed in alphabetical order.

Doctor's Data

3755 Illinois Avenue
St. Charles, IL 60174
Tel: 800-323-2784
www.doctorsdata.com

Great Smokies Diagnostic Laboratories

63 Zillicoa Street
Asheville, NC 28801
Tel: 800-522-4762
www.gsdl.com

MetaMetrix Clinical Laboratories

4855 Peachtree Ind. Blvd., Suite 201
Norcross, GA 30092
Tel: 800-221-4640
www.metametrix.com

Heavy metal tests for lead, cadmium, mercury, aluminum, and arsenic among others are not very expensive and are well worth the investment. It's best to work with a healthcare provider who is well versed in dealing with heavy metal toxicity, who will recommend many of the supplements discussed in this guide.

Testing for pesticides and solvents is more expensive. However, it is certainly worthwhile with a chronic illness that has not responded very well to many types of treatment including conventional, alternative, or integrative treatments. Once again, it is best to work with a professional with experience in getting rid of these xenobiotics and who will also recommend many of the supplements discussed in this guide.

DETOX DIET GROCERY LIST

VEGETABLES*

- Alfafa sprouts
- Arugula
- Artichokes
- Asparagus
- Bean sprouts
- Bell peppers (red, green, or yellow)
- Beets
- Bok choy
- Broccoli
- Brussels sprouts
- Cabbage (red or white)
- Carrots
- Cauliflower
- Celery
- Chickory
- Cucumbers
- Dandelion greens
- Eggplant
- Green beans
- Hot peppers
- Jicama
- Kale
- Leeks
- Lettuce (all types)
- Mushrooms
- Okra
- Onions
- Parsley
- Radishes
- Snow peas
- Spinach
- Watercress
- Water chestnuts
- Yellow squash
- Zucchini

As many and as much as you like.

FRUITS

- ❑ Apples
- ❑ Apricots
- ❑ Bananas
- ❑ Blackberries
- ❑ Boysenberries
- ❑ Cantaloupes
- ❑ Cherries
- ❑ Figs, fresh
- ❑ Grapes
- ❑ Grapefruits
- ❑ Grapefruit juice
- ❑ Guavas
- ❑ Honeydew melons
- ❑ Kiwi fruits
- ❑ Kumquats
- ❑ Lemons
- ❑ Mandarin oranges
- ❑ Mangoes
- ❑ Nectarines
- ❑ Nectars
- ❑ Oranges
- ❑ Papayas
- ❑ Passion fruits
- ❑ Peaches
- ❑ Pears
- ❑ Pineapples
- ❑ Plums
- ❑ Pomegranates
- ❑ Prunes
- ❑ Raspberries
- ❑ Strawberries

SELECTED
REFERENCES

Aggarwal BB, Takada Y, Oommen OV. From chemo-prevention to chemotherapy: common targets and common goals. *Expert Opinion in Investigative Drugs,* 2004;13(10):1327–38.

Anderson N, Benoist A. *Your Health & Your House: A Resource Guide.* New Canaan, Conn.: 1994.

American Heart Association. Air pollution, heart disease and stroke. January 16, 2005. http://www.americanheart.org/presenter.jhtml?identifier=4419

Babal K. *Good Digestion.* Burnaby, B.C.: Alive Publishing Group, 2000.

Crowe SE, Perdue MH. Gastrointestinal food hypersensitivity: Basic mechanisms of pathophysiology. *Gastroenterology,* 1992;103(3):1075–1095.

DDT. *Wikipedia—The Free Encyclopedia.* The Wikipedia Foundation, January 13, 2005. http://en.wikipedia.org/wiki/DDT

Deleve L, Kaplowitz N. Glutathione metabolism and its role in hepatotoxicity. *Pharmcology and Therapeutics,* 1991;52:287–305.

Furlong JH. Detoxification–a clinical perspective. *Quarterly Review of Natural Medicine,* 1997;Fall:243–252.

Gibson GG. Detoxication mechanisms and the role of nutrition. In: Tarcher AB (ed), *Principles and Practice of Environmental Medicine,* New York: Plenum, 1992, p 139–158.

Gormley J. Of spirits in the toxified world. *Better Nutrition,* 2001, 63(3):12.

Gormley J. Garlic and detox. *Better Nutrition,* 2000; 62(10):16.

Gormley J. Ayurveda and the science of un-toxification. *Better Nutrition,* 1997, 59(1):32.

Gursche S. *Encyclopedia of Natural Healing.* Burnaby, B.C.: Alive Publishing Group, 1997.

Haas E, Chace D, Haas EM. *The New Detox Diet: The Complete Guide for Lifelong Vitality With Recipes, Menus, and Detox Plans.* Berkeley, CA: Celestial Arts, 2004.

Hazardous incinerators. *Science News* 1993;143:334.

Kelly GS. Clinical applications of N-acetylcysteine. *Alternative Medicine Review,* 1998;3(2):114–126.

Laekeman G, De Coster S, De Meyer K. St. Mary's Thistle: an overview. *Journal of Pharmacology (Belgium),* 2003;58(1):28–31.

Lieberman S, Bruning N. *The Real Vitamin & Mineral Book* (3rd Edition). New York: Avery/Penguin-Putnam, 2003.

Milk Thistle. *Alternative Medicine Review* 1999;4(4): 272–274.

Page, LR. *Detoxification—All You Need to Know to Recharge, Renew and Rejuvenate Your Body, Mind and Spirit.* Sarasota, FL: Bookworld Services, 1998.

Parke DV. Nutritional requirements for detoxication of environmental chemicals. *Food Additives and Contaminants* 1991;8(3):381–96.

Roger F. Air pollutants may worsen allergies. *Medical Tribune* 1993;May 27:9.

Rogers AE. Diet and toxicity of chemicals. *The Journal of Nutritional Biochemistry* 1991;2:579–593.

Singh RP, Agarwal R. Flavonoid antioxidant silymarin and skin cancer. Antioxidants and Redox Signaling 2002 Aug;4(4):655–663.

Weisenburger DD. Human health effects of agrichemical use. *Human Pathology ,* 1993;24(6):571–576.

Whorton JC. *Inner Hygiene: Constipation and the Pursuit of Health in Modern Society.* New York: Oxford University Press, 2000.

Woodham A, Peters D. *Encyclopedia of Healing Therapies.* New York: DK Publishing, 1997.

OTHER BOOKS
AND RESOURCES

GreatLife Magazine
Consumer magazine with articles on vitamins, minerals, herbs, and foods.
Available for free at many health and natural food stores.

Let's Live Magazine
Consumer magazine with emphasis on the health benefits of vitamins, minerals, and herbs.
Customer service:
1-800-676-4333
P.O. Box 74908
Los Angeles, CA 90004
Subscriptions: 12 issues per year, $19.95 in the U.S.; $31.95 outside the U.S.

Physical Magazine
Magazine oriented to body builders and other serious athletes.
Customer service:
1-800-676-4333
P.O. Box 74908
Los Angeles, CA 90004
Subscriptions: 12 issues per year, $19.95 in the U.S.; $31.95 outside the U.S.

The Nutrition Reporter™ newsletter
Monthly newsletter that summarizes recent medical research on vitamins, minerals, and herbs.
Customer service:
P.O. Box 30246
Tucson, AZ 85751-0246
e-mail: jack@thenutritionreporter.com
www.nutritionreporter.com
Subscriptions: $26 per year (12 issues) in the U.S.; $32 U.S. or $48 CNC for Canada; $38 for other countries

Dr. Shari Lieberman's E-Newsletter

This free newsletter (available at www.drshari.net) reviews the current scientific literature in the field of nutrition and related fields so you can take charge of your health and well-being. Dr. Lieberman's website also features a library of research and scientific presentations.

INDEX

Acetaminophen, 42, 52, 56
Acidophilus, 60, 62–63
AGE, 52
Aged garlic extract. See
 AGE.
AIBR Scientific Reviews, 47
Air fresheners, 71
Air pollution, 10–12
ALA. See Alpha lipoic acid.
Alcohol, 21, 48
Aldrin, 4
Allium sativum. See Garlic.
Alpha lipoic acid, 16, 41,
 43–44, 75
Amanita mushrooms, 47, 53
American Journal of
 Clinical Nutrition, 37
Amine oxidase system, 14
Anderson, James W., 28
Anderson, Nina, 3
Ansari, R.A., 56
Antioxidants, 26–35, 46–47
Antiperspirants, 72
Archives of Internal
 Medicine, 42
Asbestos, 72
Ascorbic acid. See Vitamin
 C.
Assyria, 51
Ayurvedic medicine, 53–59

Babal, Ken, 19
Bahupatra niruri. See
 Phyllanthus amarus.
Benzopyrene, 37
Berkson, Burt, 34
Beta-carotene, 29, 30
Better Nutrition, 49
Bioflavonoids, 47
Biological contaminants, 10
Biotin, 34
Blood glucose. See Blood
 sugar.
Blood sugar, 61
Bottles, plastic, 67
Bowel movements, 20

Brains, 56
Breecher, Maury M., 28

Cadmium, 43
Caffeine, 21
Cancer, 36–38, 42, 52
Candida albicans, 64
Carbohydrates, 61
Carbon tetrachloride, 56
Carotenoids, 29
Cascara sagrada, 63
Cassidy, Aedin, 36
Cell membranes and milk
 thistle, 48–49
Chandler, R., 56–57
Chelation, 43
Chemical contaminants
 from indoor sources,
 9–10
 from outdoor sources, 10
Chemical poisoning, 56
Chlordane, 4
Chlorine bleach, 71
Cholesterol, 61
Choline, 34
Circulatory system, 18
Cleaning supplies, 71
Clothing, 72
Cobalamin. See Vitamin B_{12}.
Coleridge, Samuel Taylor,
 12
Colors, 22
Constipation, 61–64
Consumer Reports, 66, 69,
 70
Contaminants, 9–10
Cosmetics, 72
Culturelle, 63
Cyanocobalamin. See
 Vitamin B_{12}.
Cytochrome P450 mono-
 oxygenase system. See
 P450 detoxification
 system.

Dandelion, 22

DDT, 4, 7, 23
Death cap mushroom. See
    Amanita mushrooms.
Detox diet, 18–25
Detoxification, 1–2, 3–17,
    18–25, 26–35, 36–40,
    41–44, 45–50, 51–59,
    60–64, 65–73, 74–77,
    79–81, 82–83
    antioxidants and, 26–34
    daily program for, 74–77
    diet for, 18–25, 82–83
    enzymes and, 14
    experience, 76–77
    gastrointestinal tract and,
        17
    grocery list for, 82–83
    heavier-duty program,
        75–76
    herbs for, 51–59
    influences on, 15
    need for, 3–17
    normal daily program,
        74–75
    phase I, 13–14
    phase II, 13, 15
    phytochemicals and,
        36–40
Dialyl disulfide. See Garlic.
Dieldrin, 4
Diet, 16, 18–25
    detox, 18–25
    high fiber, 15
    Western, 12
    See also Food.
Digestion, 18–19
Digestive tract, 53
Dioxin, 4–6
Disinfectants, 71
DNA, 27–28, 42
Dr. Anderson's Antioxidant,
    Antiaging Health
    Program, 28
Dry cleaning spot
    removers, 71
Duke, James A., 45, 46
Dwivedi, Y., 56
Dymock, Warden and
    Hooper, 55
Dysentery, 53

Ellagic acid, 38
Emblica officinalis, 59

Encyclopedia of Healing
    Therapies, 12
Endrin, 4
Enterohepatic circulation, 49
Environmental toxins, 3, 60
Enzymes, 14
Estrogen, 38
Exercise, 18, 22

Fats, 21
Feher, H., 48
Fever, 18
Fiber, 1–2, 17, 19–20, 39,
    61–63, 75
Field Guide to Medicinal
    Plants: Eastern and
    Central North America,
    45
Finnish baths, 76
Fires, 5
Fish, 24–25
Flavonoids, 16, 39, 47
Flax seeds, 62
Floersheim, Mr., 55
Flora, friendly, 62–64
Florastor, 63
Flourocarbon plastic, 73
Fluids, 18
Folic acid. See Vitamin B9.
Foo, L. Yeap, 57
Food, 3, 22. See also Diet.
Formaldehyde, 71–72
Foster, Steven, 45, 46
Frackelton, Mr.,
Free radicals, 26–28, 48–49
Fruits, 20–24, 40, 83
Furans, 4–5

Garlic, 51–52
    dosage, 59
    See also AGE.
Gastrointestinal tract (GI),
    13, 17, 20, 60–64
Gerschman, R., 26
Giardia infection, 53
Glucarate, 39
Glucose. See Blood sugar.
Glutathione sulf hydryl. See
    GSH.
Good Digestion, 19
Gormley, James J., 54
Grains, whole, 34
Green drinks, 60–64, 74

Greenpeace, 5
GSH, 16, 41–44, 52, 76
Guar gum, 62

Hair dyes, 72
Harman, Denham, 26
HDPE plastic, 67
*Healing Benefits of Garlic,
    The,* 51
Health, cornerstones of, 19
Heavy metals. See Metals,
    heavy.
Heinerman, John, 51
Hepatitis B, 58
Heptachlor, 4
Herbal detoxifiers, other,
    51–59
Herbal Tonic Therapies, 45,
    46, 49
Herbs, 21, 40, 53–59
Hexachlorobenzene, 4
Hoffmann, David, 46, 47
HVAC, 9

Immune system, 44
Indian Materia Medica, 57
Indoles, 38
Indoor air quality, 8–10
Inositol, 33–34
Insecticides, 7, 73
Isoflavones, 36–37

Janson, Michael, 32
*Japananese Journal of
    Pharmacology,* 52
Jayaram, Mr., 58
*Journal of Applied
    Nutrition,* 23
Juicing, 20

Kelp, 60
Khanum, F., 52
Kidneys, 13

Leon, 22
L-glutamine, 62
Leaky gut syndrome, 62
Leukotrienes, 49
Lignans, 37–38
Lipofuscins, 27
Lipoic acid. See Alpha
    lipoic acid.
Lipolysis, 76

Lipophilic, 13
Liver, 13, 20, 45, 46, 48, 51,
    53–54, 55–57
  disease, 45
  milk thistle and, 46, 48
  Picrorhiza kuroa and,
    55–56
  toxicity, 45
Lungs, 13
Lymphatic system, 18

McCaleb, Rob, 48
Mercury, 43
Metals, heavy, 23, 44, 60,
    72, 80–81
  testing for, 80–81
Milk thistle, 16, 45–50, 60, 74
  antioxidant properties,
    46–47
  as a free-radical
    scavenger, 48–49
  cell membranes and,
    48–49
  dosages, 49–50
  enterohepatic circulation
    and, 49
  known compounds of, 46
  liver and, 46
Mirex, 4
Mold cleaners, 71
Monoterpenes, 39
Mothballs, 71
Mowrey, Daniel B., 45, 46, 49
Mukhtar, Hasan, 37
Munday, R & C.M., 52
Murray, Frank, 47, 49
Mushrooms, 47, 51

N-acetylcysteine (NAC), 16,
    41–44, 75
Nadkarni, K.M., 57
Natural Pharmacy, 31
Nature vs anti-nature, 15
New Holistic Herbal, The,
    46
NHANES, 40
Niacin. See Vitamin B$_3$.
Nitrogen oxides, 11–12
NMVOCs, 11
Non-methane volatile
    organic compounds.
    See NMVOCs.
Nutrients, 14–15, 19

Nutrition and Cancer, 52
Nutrition. *See* Diet.
Nutritional supplements.
    See Supplements.

Oat bran, 62
Omega-3 fatty acids, 24
Organic produce, 23–24
Oven cleaners, 71
Oxidation, 27
Oxygen, 28
Ozone, 11

P450 detoxification system,
    14, 16–17
Pandey, V.N., 56
Pantothenic acid. *See*
    Vitamin B$_5$.
Papyrus Ebers, 1
Paracetamol overdose, 56
Parasites, 56, 65–66
PCBs, 4–6, 23, 66
Pectin, 62
Pernicious anemia, 33
Persistent organic
    pollutants. *See* POPs.
Personal-care products, 72
Pesticides, 23, 56, 73, 79
PET bottles. *See*
    Polyethylene bottles.
Phyllanthus amarus, 57–58
    components, 58
    dosage, 59
    how it works, 58
Phytochemicals, 36–40, 57,
    60, 75
Phytonadione. *See* Vitamin
    K.
Picrorhiza kurroa, 16, 53,
    55–57
    acetominophen overdose
        and, 56
    chemical poisoning and,
        56
    components, 55
    dosage, 59
    how it works, 57
    parasites and 56
Plant foods, 38–40
Plasmodium berghei, 56
Plastics, 72
Pollution, 8–12
    air, 10–12

    household, 8–10
Polyacetylene, 37
Polychlorinated biphenyls.
    See PCBs.
Polyethylene, 72
    bottles, 67
Polyphenols, 37
Polyvinyl chloride, 72
POPs, 3–4
Potter, John, 38
Prasad, Kedar, 29
Precursor, 43
Proteins, 24
Pryor, William A., 27
Psyllium, 62
Pyridoxine. *See* Vitamin B$_6$.

QR, 52
Quercetin, 39
Quicksilver. *See* Mercury.
Quinone reductase. *See* QR.

Rastogi, R., 55
Rest, 21
Riboflavin. *See* Vitamin B$_2$.
Ricebran, 62
*Rime of the Ancient
    Mariner,* 12

Saccharomyces boulardii.
    See Florastor.
Salads, 21
Saraswat, B., 56
Saturday Night Live, 2
Saunas, 76
Science, 12
Seaweed, 60
Selenium, 30
Senna, 63
Serum tests, 78–81
Shichi, Dr., 51
Sick building syndrome,
    8–10
    causes, 8–10
Silybum marianum. See
    Milk thistle.
Silymarin, 45–50, 74. *See
    also* Milk Thistle.
Singh, V., 56
Skin, 13
Sleep, 21
Soda, 21
Solvents, 79

Soy, 37
Spices, 21, 40
Spirulina, 60–61
Sterols, 37
Stuart Oil Shale Project, 5
Sugar, 20, 21. *See also*
   Blood sugar.
Sulforaphanes, 39
Sumioka, I., 52
Supper green drinks,
   60–64, 74
Supplements, 15
   for constipation, 62–64
   recommended levels of,
   44, 59
   when to consider, 44
Sweeteners, 21

Tea, herbal, 21–22, 62
Terminalia bellerica, 59
Terminalia chebula, 59
Testing, 79–81
Thiamine. *See* Vitamin B_1.
Thyagarajan, S.P., 58
Tocopderls, 30
Toxaphene, 4, 5
Toxins, 3–17, 18–25, 26–35,
   36–40, 41–44, 45–50,
   51–59, 60–64, 65–73,
   74–77, 79–81
   diet to purge, 18–25
   reducing, 12–13
Triphala, 58–59, 63
   dosage, 59
Trowell, 1
Tyler, Varro, 46

United Nations, 5
United Nations Environment
   Programme Intergov-
   ernmental Negotiating
   Committee for a Treaty
   on Persistent Organic
   Pollutants, 4
Unitoxification, 53–54
Urea-formaldehyde plastic
   resins, 73
U.S. Environmental Protec-
   tion Agency, 7–8, 11–12

Vegetables, 16, 20–24, 40,
   82

Ventilation, inadequate, 8–9
Vinyl chloride, 72
Vitamin A, 30–31
Vitamin B complex, 26–35,
   74
Vitamin B_1, 31
Vitamin B_2, 31
Vitamin B_3, 31–32
Vitamin B_5, 32
Vitamin B_6, 32–33
Vitamin B_9, 33
Vitamin B_{12}, 33
Vitamin C, 30–31, 43
Vitamin E, 30, 43, 47
Vitamin Revolution, 32
Vitamins, multi-, 74
VOCs, 7–9, 10–11, 56
Vogel, G., 47
Volatile organic
   compounds. *See* VOCs.

Waste elimination, 19
Water, 12, 21–22, 63, 65–70
   bottled, 66–67
   mineral, 67–68
   naturally sparkling, 69
   purification systems,
   68–70
   purified, 68
   sodas and seltzer, 68
   tap, 65–66
   types, 67–68
Water Quality Association,
   70
Weather, 54
Wheat bran, 62
Wheat grass, 60–61
Wikipedia, 7
Williams, Roger J., 32
Wong, Herbert, 57
World Health Organization,
   8, 12
Worms, 53

Xenobiotics, 3, 15–16, 29,
   44, 49, 61–62, 71, 76,
   79–81
Xenohormones, 38

Your Health & Your House, 3

Zhao, Dr., 51